C
A G ... to im... ... for
Healthcare Professionals

Second Edition

Rob McSherry
RGN, DipN (Lon), BSc (Hons), MSc, PGCE, RT
Principal Lecturer, Practice Development
School of Health and Social Care, University of Teesside
Middlesbrough

and

Paddy Pearce
RGN, BSc (Hons), MSc
Head of Healthcare Governance
Hambleton and Richmondshire Primary Care Trust
Thirsk, North Yorkshire

with a contribution by

John Tingle
BA (Law Hons), MEd, Barrister
Reader in Health Law
Director of the Centre for Health Law
Nottingham Trent University, Nottingham

Blackwell
Publishing

Blackwell Publishing editorial offices:
Blackwell Publishing Ltd, 9600 Garsington Road, Oxford OX4 2DQ, UK
Tel: +44 (0)1865 776868
Blackwell Publishing Inc., 350 Main Street, Malden, MA 02148-5020, USA
Tel: +1 781 388 8250
Blackwell Publishing Asia Pty Ltd, 550 Swanston Street, Carlton, Victoria 3053, Australia
Tel: +61 (0)3 8359 1011

First edition published 2002 by Blackwell Publishing
Second edition published 2007

ISBN-10: 1-4051-3920-X
ISBN-13: 978-1-4051-3920-5

Library of Congress Cataloging-in-Publication Data
McSherry, Robert.
Clinical governance: a guide to implementation for healthcare professionals/Rob
McSherry and Paddy Pearce, with a contribution by John Tingle. – 2nd ed.
p. ; cm.
Includes bibliographical references and index.
ISBN-13: 978-1-4051-3920-5 (pbk.: alk. paper)
ISBN-10: 1-4051-3920-X (pbk.: alk. paper)
1. Medical care–Quality control. 2. Medical audit. 3. Clinical competence.
I. Pearce, Paddy. II. Tingle, John. III. Title.
[DNLM: 1. State Medicine–standards. 2. Clinical Medicine–standards. 3. Medical
Audit. 4. Patient Care Management–standards. 5. Quality Assurance, Health Care.
W 225 FA1 M389c 2006]
RA399.A1 M375 2006
362.1068–dc22
2006019513

A catalogue record for this title is available from the British Library

Set in 10/12.5pt Sabon
by Graphicraft Limited, Hong Kong
Printed and bound in Singapore
by Markono Print Media Pte Ltd

The publisher's policy is to use permanent paper from mills that operate a sustainable forestry
policy, and which has been manufactured from pulp processed using acid-free and elementary
chlorine-free practices. Furthermore, the publisher ensures that the text paper and cover board
used have met acceptable environmental accreditation standards.

For further information on Blackwell Publishing, visit our website:
www.blackwellpublishing.com

Contents

Foreword

In 1998, the Chief Medical Officer, Sir Liam Donaldson, described clinical governance as a 'ten-year journey'. As the authors of this book demonstrate eloquently, much has been achieved in the intervening eight years – but a great deal still needs to be done if the potential of clinical governance is to be fully realised and if its aspirations of uniform excellence in care are to be achieved.

With the public sector reform agenda gathering pace, with major structural reorganisation within the NHS in England a reality and with the advent of a competitive provider market place in health care, it is timely to pause and reflect not only on what has been achieved, but upon the challenges that now confront healthcare professionals and the distinctive contribution that clinical governance can make in meeting these challenges.

First and foremost, it is important to emphasise that there is no contradiction between the profound system reform that is demanded by *A Patient-Led NHS* and clinical governance. From the outset clinical governance has had two foci. The first is upon the reliability and safety of existing provision. The second has always been upon the transformation that is necessary in the culture, models, patterns and locations of NHS care if services are to be responsive to the emergent needs of a rapidly changing society, the rising expectations of individual citizens and the imperative of promoting equity in health and well being – that most basic of human rights.

Clinical governance is not, and has never been, an end in itself. Alongside effective financial and general management it is one essential means to the promotion of sustained quality in the care provided by individual healthcare staff, by teams, by organisations and by a co-ordinated and coherent local health (and social care) system. It is a primary means through which NHS organisations are assured that they are discharging a number of their key statutory duties, foremost amongst which are the duty of 'quality' and the duty of 'patient and public involvement'. Properly understood and implemented, clinical governance also plays a significant role in the discharge of the overall 'duty of care' (to staff and patients alike), in information and research governance and it provides a key focus through which the duty of 'partnership' is given concrete expression via the co-ordinated management of the patient pathway across organisational boundaries and sectoral frontiers.

As a result, clinical governance systems, processes and outcomes have a pivotal role in generating the evidence that underpins a Board's assurance that the organisation is compliant with the core elements of *Standards for Better Health*, and that it is purposefully engaged with and making progress in relation to the developmental standards. In this way clinical governance has a profound impact upon the way in that an organisation's performance will be rated through the Healthcare Commission's 'Annual Healthcheck'.

Over the last few years I have had the privilege to work with thousands of those who provide front-line care, who manage services and who govern NHS organisations. Time and again I have been inspired by their individual passion and their sustained commitment – and, like them, I have often felt frustrated that despite all of this endeavour far too often the system still fails some of the sick and most vulnerable members of our society. This remains the great challenge for clinical governance – to sustain individual commitment and to harness it in the purposeful, aligned and sustained pursuit of excellence.

I suspect that a sustained emphasis upon the elements of clinical governance will be necessary, not just for the 'last two years' of a ten-year journey but over the next decade. Over this period we must all wrestle with and respond to a pluralist and competitive health and social care market place in which individual choice, payment by results, technological innovation and genetic advances all conspire to challenge historically based assumptions about NHS provision. In the landscape of care that emerges over the next few years there will be significant shifts in activity, in resources and in staffing from hospital to locality and community-based provision. New forms of organisation will emerge to provide much of this PCT-commissioned care, so that all NHS staff will need to work in effective collaborative partnerships with staff from the private and independent sectors and with those from social care – providing even greater challenges to the delivery of a coherent and managed care pathway.

And yet, for all of this change, many of the key front-line building blocks of care must be nurtured and sustained, albeit in sometimes unfamiliar contexts or settings. Like my late friend and colleague, Ian Kramer, one of England's foremost 'expert patients', I am an NHS baby and, like him, I expect that I will die in receipt of NHS care. When that time comes, I trust that I will be cared for by someone who has fully embraced the clinical governance principles set out in this book. They reminds us that, in the final analysis, like most forms of excellence in human endeavour, clinical governance is an expression of that value-based, scientifically informed artistry that has long been exemplified by the dedicated and expert healthcare professional.

Paul Anthony Stanton
Director of Board Development
Clinical Governance Support Team

Preface

We are delighted to present this second edition of *Clinical Governance: A Guide to Implementation for Healthcare Professionals*. In this edition we have retained many of the key features of the original text, particularly with regard to:

- The evolution of clinical governance
- What clinical governance is
- What the key components of clinical governance are
- The legal implications of clinical governance
- The barriers to implementing clinical governance in clinical practice

We aim to address the above by using reflective questions, activities and case studies taken from today's healthcare services. We have developed the original theme of clinical governance and present a more integrated approach to achieving it. The information contained in the book is based upon a combination of the authors' clinical experience, knowledge and understanding of clinical governance and information derived from reading and reviewing the literature.

Rob McSherry
Paddy Pearce

Dedication

To my late parents Wilfred and Dorothy McSherry who I miss dearly. You are always in my thoughts and would have been proud to share this with me.

Rob McSherry

Chapter 1

Introduction and Background: Clinical Governance and the National Health Service

Rob McSherry and Paddy Pearce

Introduction

This chapter briefly describes the term 'clinical governance', identifying the key drivers for its inauguration into the National Health Service. The term 'clinical governance' became prominent following the publication of New Labour's first White Paper on health, *The New NHS: Modern, Dependable* (Department of Health 1997). Within this document the government sets out its agenda of modernising the National Health Service (NHS) by focusing on quality improvements. Clinical quality is rightfully assigned centre stage by 'placing duties and expectation on local health-care organisations as well as individuals' (DH 1997, p. 34) to provide clinical excellence. The vehicle for delivering clinical quality is termed 'clinical governance', which 'is being put in place in order to tackle the wide differences in the quality of care throughout the country, as well as help to address public concern about well-publicised cases of poor professional performance' (King's Fund 1999, p. 1). We believe a complicated series of factors have contributed to the development of the clinical governance agenda within healthcare. These can be distilled and categorised into three main drivers: political, professional and public demands, all attempting to revive a failing NHS and improve the quality of care that the public should rightfully expect in a modern society (McSherry 2004).

Background

Why the need for clinical governance?

The literature offered by Harvey (1998), Swage (1998) and Scally and Donaldson (1998) attributes the need for clinical governance to a decline in the standards and quality of healthcare provision, a point reinforced by the government: 'A series of well publicised lapses in quality have prompted doubts in the minds of patients about the overall standard of care they may receive' (DH 1997, p. 5). Upon reviewing the early literature (Donaldson & Halligan 2001) on clinical governance we noted that a key question had not been fully addressed about why there was a perception in the decline of standards and quality. Possible reasons for this perception could be attributed to the following. First, healthcare professionals and the public are better informed and educated, and are interested in health-related issues, thus demanding high quality service provision. Second, quality and clinical standards have taken a back seat to other financial and resource management issues. Third, political and societal changes have led to a consumerist society where patients and their carers expect to choose where and when they access healthcare. Fourth, high quality care is seen as a prerequisite. Within this chapter it is our intention to explore the factors that may have contributed to the introduction of clinical governance.

Activity 1.1: Reflective question

Write down the factors that you feel may have led to the introduction of clinical governance.

Read on and compare your answers with the findings at the end of the chapter.

No single factor has led to the government's current position regarding modernisation, currently referred to as 'system reform'. We argue that patients' and carers' expectations of and demands on healthcare professionals have increased significantly over the past decade. In the 1980s and early 1990s public awareness of healthcare provision was increased through targeted facilitation by the publication of significant documents, notably The Patient's Charter (1992) and The Citizen's Charter (1993), both of which were readily and freely made available to the public. On the one hand, these Charters may have increased patients' and carers' expectations of healthcare, by offering information about certain rights to care, but on the other hand, the responsibilities of the patients to use these rights in a responsible way have been overused, resulting in higher demands for care and services in an already busy organisation. Perhaps this has arisen because the original documents failed to emphasise the need to exercise their rights prudently. Between the 1990s and 2005 we have seen a huge emphasis placed on patient and public involvement (PPI) in the planning, delivery and quality assessment of care. Public and patient involvement has been targeted at both a national and local level both directly and indirectly through the establishment of Patient Advisory and Liaison Services (DH 2000a) within every NHS organisation. Nationally we have witnessed the establishment of the Commission for Patient and Public Involvement (DH 2003), resulting in the creation of Patient and Public User Involvement Fora, and the development of the Overview and Scrutiny Committees for Health (HMSO 2002) with the sole purpose of seeking and representing public opinion on the quality of healthcare.

In addition, other contributing factors such as changes in health policy, demographic changes, increased patient dependency, changes in healthcare delivery systems, trends towards greater access to healthcare information, advances in health technology, increased media coverage of healthcare and rising numbers of complaints going to litigation have influenced the need for a unified approach to providing and assuring clinical quality via clinical governance (McNeil 1998). These will now be debated in further detail under three broad headings (Figure 1.1): political, public and professional.

Political

Political drivers for governance should be viewed with both a capital 'P' and small 'p'. The capital 'P' refers to those drivers resulting directly from government and policy. The small 'p' relates to organisational and personal factors that influence change and policy decision-making at a local level, a view held by Jarrold (2005):

> 'politics with a small p makes the world go round. Getting things done, seeking support, building alliances, compromising – that's all politics, and inescapable and natural.' (p. 35)

The challenge for healthcare professionals is translating policy into practice and keeping up-to-date with changes in healthcare policy.

Changes in health policy

In brief, the NHS was established in 1948 following the passing of the National Health Services Act 1946 which committed the government at the time to financially funding a health service 'which rested on the principles of collectivism, comprehensiveness, equality and universality' (Allsop 1984, p. 12). The politicians at the time thought that by addressing the healthcare needs of the public, this would subsequently reduce the amount of money required to maintain the NHS, the assumption being that disease could be controlled. However, this was not the case. NHS activity spiralled, resulting in uncontrollable year-on-year expenditure to

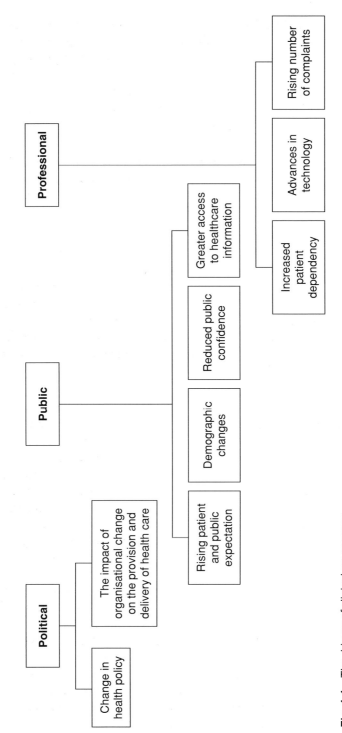

Fig. 1.1 The drivers of clinical governance.

meet the rise in public demand for healthcare. In an attempt to manage this trend, the government introduced the principles of general management via the NHS Griffiths Report (Griffiths 1983). The philosophy of general management was that of developing efficiency and effectiveness of services. The rationale behind this report was to provide services that addressed healthcare needs (effectiveness) within optimal resource allocation (efficiency). It recommended:

> 'that general managers should be appointed at all levels in the NHS to provide leadership, introduce a continual search for change and cost improvement, motivate staff and develop a more dynamic management approach.' (Ham 1986, p. 33)

Key organisational processes were identified as missing in the report:

> 'Absence of this general management support means that there is no driving force seeking and accepting direct and personal responsibility for developing management plans, securing their implementation and monitoring actual achievement. It means that the process of devolution of responsibility, including discharging responsibility to units, is far too slow.' (Griffiths 1983, p. 12)

This approach, whilst noble at the time, was concerned with organisational, managerial and financial aspects of the NHS, to the detriment of other important issues such as clinical quality. This style of management further evolved with the introduction of the White Paper *Working for Patients* (1989), culminating in the development of a 'market forces' approach to the organisation and delivery of healthcare services by the creation of a purchaser and provider split. Health authorities and general practitioner fund holders were allocated resources (finances) to purchase care for their local population at the best price. The purchaser/provider split in England and Wales was terminated by the New Labour Government and replaced by Primary Care Groups (PCGs). The PCGs would later evolve into Primary Care Trusts, becoming responsible for commissioning primary and secondary care (Baggott 2004, p. 120). These imbalances led to the introduction of the White Papers *The New NHS: Modern, Dependable* (DH 1997) and *Quality in the New NHS* (DH 1998a), which put clinical quality on a par with organisational, managerial and financial aspects of healthcare via 'clinical governance' – a framework 'which is viewed positively by many healthcare professionals as an ambitious shift of focus by the current government in moving away from finance to quality' (McSherry & Haddock 1999, p. 114). This approach to providing healthcare services places a statutory duty on matching moral responsibilities with managers' and clinicians' responsibilities/duties more closely in assuring clinical and non-clinical quality. The impact of these reforms (DH 1989, 1997, 1998) has enhanced public awareness and expectations of the NHS, placing a strong emphasis on achieving clinical quality through restructuring and changing of services.

The impact of organisational change on the provision and delivery of healthcare

With an increase in the number of patients admitted with multiple needs, healthcare organisations have had to change their pattern of care delivery in order to accommodate this growing need, leading to the development of acute medical and surgical assessment units, pre-operative assessment units, multiple needs and rehabilitation units, and acute mental health assessment units. Latterly we have witnessed an increase in the development of services dedicated to maintain individuals in the community, such as Mental Health Crisis Intervention Teams (DH 2001) and the management of patients with long-term conditions (e.g. diabetes and chronic obstructive pulmonary disease). This style of service provision is about optimising the use of acute and community beds by encouraging collaborative working between primary and secondary care in the management and maintenance of the patient in the most appropriate setting. An example of this would be the shared management of patients who have diabetes, where the care is shared between the GP and consultant endocrinologist with the backing of the diabetic team (diabetes nurse specialist, dietitian, podiatrist, ophthalmologist and pharmacist). Initiatives such as hospital-at-home schemes (where possible maintaining the patient in his or her own home) are beginning to be developed, along with public and private sector partnerships (for example, acute illness is managed in hospital, and rehabilitation is continued in a private nursing home until the patient is ready for discharge).

The contributing and reinforcing factors that necessitated these innovations could be attributed to the reduction in junior doctors' hours (DH 1998b) and the possible effects of the European Working Time Directive (DH 2004), culminating in the development of nurse practitioners particularly in highly busy areas such as acute medical admissions and accident and emergency departments. This concept was reinforced recently by the introduction of nurse consultants and therapists (McSherry & Johnson 2005) in order to accommodate the increasing demands for healthcare owing to the increase in the life expectancy of people with greater healthcare needs. These changes to healthcare delivery are directed towards enhancing the quality of care and in raising public confidence.

Public

The public have contributed significantly towards the introduction of clinical governance and its ongoing development both directly and indirectly. The ways in which the public have an effect vary in nature, from rising expectations to changes in demography.

Rising patient and public expectations and involvement

The Patient's Charter (1992) *Raising the Standards* was distributed to all householders in the United Kingdom (UK) and detailed patients' and carers' rights to healthcare. The main principles behind this charter were that of informing and empowering patients and this led to patients being viewed as consumers of healthcare. As consumers, they are entitled to certain rights and standards of care. These standards included the right to be registered with a general practitioner, to have a named consultant and qualified nurse as an in-patient, and the right to be seen within thirty minutes of any specified appointment time with a healthcare practitioner. The Patient's Charter reinforced the aims of The Citizen's Charter (1993) by empowering the individual to become actively involved in the delivery of health services by the granting of certain rights. This style of healthcare delivery was unique, as previously patients tended to be seen as passive recipients of often paternalistic methods of providing care ('the doctor knows best').

However, the benefits of these Charters have been variable: some individuals (both the public and healthcare professionals) are unaware of how they can be used to promote raised standards, while in contrast many other patients/carers are much more aware and informed of certain rights to treatments and healthcare interventions. In general, the majority of healthcare professionals have taken up and accepted the challenges posed by these Charters in improving the delivery and organisation of healthcare. This can be evidenced by reviewing outpatient waiting time, hospital league tables and the introduction of the named qualified nurse within inpatient settings. It could be argued that The Patient's Charter has led to a public that are more questioning about their rights and expectations of healthcare: What is the problem? How will the condition be treated? What are the alternatives? What are the potential risks and benefits of all treatment options? These are genuine concerns that need addressing.

While raising awareness and expectations of healthcare services has had benefits, a limitation of The Patient's Charter is that it has also created a demand which at times has been difficult to satisfy for many healthcare trusts. For example, to have a named qualified nurse assess, plan, implement and evaluate care from admission to discharge was impractical and overestimated. Similarly it is sometimes difficult for a consultant to see all his or her outpatient attendees personally on every visit. The consequence of raising expectations which are not achievable results in dissatisfaction with services and a higher incidence of complaints. The principles behind the Charters are plausible providing the services are resourced sufficiently. Furthermore the publication of waiting times and league tables has highlighted inequalities in the provision of healthcare across the nation. For example, access to services such as day case surgery can be variable according to region or demographic status of the local population.

League tables have a failing in that on their own they do not provide the public with background information on local community health trends or the availability of healthcare services for individual trusts, hence the disparity of service provision between trusts. It could be the case that it may be inappropriate to perform day case surgery for hernia repairs in a hospital situated in a rural area with a large elderly population because of accessibility of services and appropriateness of the surgery to the patients' needs. This is more evident in society today with an ever increasing elderly population with multi-complex physical, social and psychological needs which place yet further demands on the health service, making The Patient's Charter standards even more difficult to achieve.

Since the introduction of clinical governance through the White Paper (DH 1997) we have seen a dramatic shift from limited patient and public involvement to a statutory requirement for quality (HMSO 2003). This is evident by the publication of the Freedom of Information Act (DH 2000c) and the Patient and Public Fora (DH 2003). These Acts and policy changes encourage NHS organisations to systematically involve the patient and users in making decisions about the development, provision and experience of the services they have accessed. The Patient and Public Fora (DH 2003) and Patient Advisory Liaison Services (PALS) are two national examples of the government's commitment to improving services for the public. A key outcome of the government's health polices is placing patients at the heart of service development, delivery and evaluation. PPI is critical in a modern consumerist society in ensuring that services are truly representative and reflective of patient and public needs. This is important in light of changes in demography and dependency.

Demographic changes

Public health policy and findings from national surveys (National Statistics 2004) reiterate the government's findings in *Health of the Nation* (DH 1991), which highlighted that life expectancy would increase along with changes in the patterns of mortality and morbidity, for example, an increased prevalence of diabetes and obesity (Press Association 2005). As a consequence of these changes the NHS needs to provide more acute, continuing care and primary care services for an increasingly elderly population and to take into account the changes in the patterns of disease and illness associated with societal change. In an attempt to reduce healthcare demands, *Health of the Nation* set targets for reducing morbidity (disease and disability trends) by concentrating upon health promotion and disease prevention, for example the reduction of strokes by the active management of high blood pressure (hypertension) and the reduction of deaths attributed to coronary heart disease by promoting healthy eating, exercise and, where necessary, the prescription of 'statins' (cholesterol lowering drugs) (DH 2000b).

Population statistics indicate there has and will continue to be a large increase in the numbers of people living to and beyond sixty-five, seventy-five and eighty-five. Longevity seems to be on the increase for all (DH 1991), reinforcing the growing trend of high-dependency patients. Longevity is not the only demographic challenge facing the future NHS; we have seen widening inequalities in health, wealth and disease. There is growing public health concern about obesity, sexual health, drug- and alcohol-related problems, all of which will lead to greater demands on the health service and its employees.

Lack of public confidence in healthcare provision due to media coverage of poor clinical practices

The media continues to play a major role in increasing patients' and carers' awareness of the NHS through the publication of clinical successes and failures, for example The Bristol Royal Infirmary Inquiry 2001 and the Shipman Inquiry 2005. The Bristol case related to consultant paediatric cardiac surgeons who were found to have a death rate for paediatric heart surgery that was significantly higher than the national average. This only became known as a result of whistle blowing (Lancet 1998). The Shipman case involved a general practitioner in Manchester who was found to have murdered many patients mainly by injecting them with an overdose of class A drugs such as morphine and diamorphine. The impact of these major failings and others has resulted in a lack of public confidence in the health service, and a concomitant rise in the number of complaints proceeding to litigation (Wilson & Tingle 1999).

Trend towards greater access to healthcare information

Advances in information technology, such as the internet, have resulted in easier access to information by the public. Individuals are able to access the same information as healthcare professionals, for example The Cochrane Library and the Department of Health website inform patients with specific information relating to their condition. This ability to access information that was perhaps previously difficult to obtain is fuelling the public's demands for and expectations of quality care. Healthcare professionals need to be aware of both these rising expectations and the implications of the Freedom of Information Act (DH 2003), which has made access to healthcare information easier. Furthermore, websites such as Doctor Foster (www.drfoster.co.uk), the National Electronic Library for Health (NeLH) (www.nelh.nhs.uk) and the Commission for Patient and Public Involvement in Health (www.cppih.org; see also DH 2003), which encourage the public to become more involved in the delivery of healthcare, reinforce the need for professionals to be aware of giving, receiving and signposting patients and carers to relevant sources of information.

Professional

Several factors are emerging that may impact on or compromise health-care professionals' accountability. These are increased patient dependency, advanced technology and the rise in litigious activities.

Increased patient dependency

The increasing number of elderly people means that patients are being admitted into acute and community hospitals with far more multi-complex physical and social problems (McSherry 1999) than ever before, requiring timely appropriate interventions from a wide range of health and social care practitioners. Such multi-disciplinary and cross agency collaborative working has resulted in significant improvements, for example the average length of stay in acute hospital following total hip replacement surgery has gone down from fourteen to seven days. A further example is in the advances in stroke care and rehabilitation and in the establishment of specialist stroke units where the evidence clearly demonstrates that recovery is better if stroke patients are managed in a specialist unit and not on an acute general medical ward (Stroke Unit Trialists' Collaboration 1998). The major effect of the rise in dependency has been the need for greater efficiency, such as minimising length of hospital stay and maintaining high levels of acute bed occupancy.

However, the shorter average length of patient stay also has consequences in that it is sometimes not possible to be as effective in discharge planning, due to staff having less planning time (particularly in complex social cases). Readmission rates have increased and more demands are being made on community nursing services, hospital-at-home schemes, and continuing and long-term care facilities, as there are more patients with complex physical and social needs requiring continued healthcare. Multi-agency or cross-sectoral professional working poses a challenge since 'clinical governance' is not easily understood, nor does it have a direct equivalent in social care.

Advances in healthcare technology

Advances in healthcare technology have made inroads in improving the quality and standards of nursing care delivery, for example, pressure-relieving equipment, moving and handling equipment, medical administration and monitoring equipment and wound care management. All have the potential for enhancing the quality of care delivered by healthcare professionals. However, credentialisation (demonstrating that staff have the knowledge, competence and skills to use the equipment safely) may be questionable. This is because it is often difficult to arrange time and resources for staff to be trained in safe equipment usage in an ever demanding and stressful clinical environment. Further, this represents a particular challenge to PCTs with regard to independent contractors – dentists, pharmacists, optometrists, etc. This should not be the case if clinical governance is implemented successfully. The pressures being placed upon healthcare professionals to deliver a high quality service based upon appropriate evidence have the potential to create a conflict between balancing efficiency and effectiveness and maintaining quality and standards. A balance cannot be achieved without adequate resourcing, government backing and some cultural change within the healthcare services.

Rising numbers of complaints going to litigation

Over the past decade there has been a huge rise in the number of formal complaints made by patients and carers about hospital and community services, proceeding to litigation. The National Heath Service Litigation Authority (NHSLA) paid out £502.9 million for clinical negligence claims in 2004–2005 compared to £422.5 million in 2003–2004 (NHSLA, www.nhsla.com/claims/). These increased costs have been attributed to:

- Increased activity levels of healthcare to deal with increased demand.
- Greater propensity to pursue a complaint to litigation.
- Increased compensation for negligence claims (so people are more likely to seek redress when something goes wrong).

It is worth noting here that the vast majority of complaints are resolved at a local level, often with clarification, explanations and an apology for when things have gone wrong. Honesty and openness are the key to dealing with complaints, as well as the development of robust mechanisms for the sharing of information to deal with issues before they become problems (McSherry 1996). Management needs to encourage a learning culture, which proactively rather than reactively responds when something goes wrong. The ultimate aim is to have a fair blame culture that encourages nurses to openly report, discuss and learn from clinical incidents or clinical complaints. In many instances complaints arise from system failures rather than the actions or omissions of individuals. Healthcare professionals need to be made aware of this situation and have the knowledge, skills, competence and confidence to deal positively with complaints.

Summary

Activity 1.1: Feedback

Factors that lead to the introduction of clinical governance can be attributed to the following:

- Changes in health policy
- The impact of organisational change on the provision and delivery of healthcare
- Rising patient and public expectations and involvement
- Demographic changes
- Lack of public confidence in healthcare provision due to media coverage of poor clinical practices
- Trend towards greater access to healthcare information
- Increased patient dependency
- Advances in healthcare technology
- Rising numbers of complaints going to litigation

A closer review of the above factors demonstrates three primary drivers for clinical governance. These originate from the 'three p' approach to clinical governance: political, professional and public.

It is clear from Activity 1.1 that there are many contributing factors that influence the introduction of clinical governance within the NHS. Undoubtedly more factors will continue to arise, reinforcing the need for clinical governance in the future. It is therefore important that organisations and individuals embrace the concept of clinical governance in the pursuit of clinical excellence as a journey. The latter can only be achieved by having an understanding of where clinical governance originated and what it means in daily clinical practice, as outlined in Chapter 2.

Key points

The reasons for introducing clinical governance into the NHS were:

- A perceived decline in clinical standards, service provision and delivery. This was reinforced by media coverage of major clinical failures, notably the Bristol and Shipman inquiries, resulting in a general lack of public confidence in the NHS.
- A more informed, consumer-orientated public with greater expectations of the NHS, this being attributed to the different charters.
- A more questioning and litigious society. A combination of political, professional and public factors that have led to the introduction of clinical governance and the pursuit of quality in the NHS.

Suggested reading

Donaldson, L.J. & Muir Grey, J.A. (1998) Clinical governance; a quality duty for health organisations. *Quality in Healthcare*, 7 (Suppl) S37–S44.

McNeil, J. (1998) Clinical governance: the whys, whats, and hows for theatre practitioners. *British Journal of Theatre Nursing*, 9 (5) 208–216.

Pickering, S. & Thompson, J. (2003) *Clinical Governance and Best Value: Meeting the Modernisation Agenda*. Churchill Livingstone, London.

References

Allsop, J. (1984) *Health Policy and The National Health Service*. Longman, London.

Baggott, R. (2004) *Health and Healthcare in Britain*, 3rd edn. Palgrave Macmillan, Basingstoke.

Department of Health (1989) White Paper: *Working for Patients*. HMSO, London.

Department of Health (1991) *Health of the Nation*. HMSO, London.

Department of Health (1992) *Raising the Standards*. HMSO, London.

Department of Health (1993) *The Citizen's Charter*. HMSO, London.

Department of Health (1997) *The New NHS: Modern and Dependable*. HMSO, London.

Department of Health (1998a) *Quality in the New NHS*. HMSO, London.

Department of Health (1998b) Reducing junior doctors' hours: continuing action to meet New Deal standards. *Health Services Circular 1998/240*. DH, London.

Department of Health (2000a) *The NHS Plan: A Plan for Investment, a Plan for Reform*. HMSO, London.

Department of Health (2000b) *National Service Framework for Coronary Heart Disease: Modern Standards and Service Models*. DH, London.

Department of Health (2000c) *Freedom of Information Act 2000.* www.dh.gov.uk/PolicyAndGuidance/FreedomOfInformation/fs/en.

Department of Health (2001) *Major Cash Boost for Mental Health Services.* Ref No. 2001/0544. www.dh.gov.uk/PublicationsAndStatistics/PressReleases/PressReleasesNotices/fs/en?CONTENT_ID=4011514&chk=dUYGu/.

Department of Health (2003) *Patient and Public Involvement Forums Go Live.* Ref No. 2003/0483. www.dh.gov.uk/PublicationsAndStatistics/PressReleases/PressReleasesNotices/fs/en?CONTENT_ID=4062851&chk=/YNcaY.

Department of Health (2004) *European Working Time Directive.* www.dh.gov.uk/PolicyAndGuidance/HumanResourcesAndTraining/Working Differently/EuropeanWorkingTimeDirective/fs/en.

Donaldson, L. & Halligan, A. (2001) Implementing clinical governance: turning vision into reality. *BMJ*, 322 (7299).

Griffiths, R. (1983) *NHS Management Enquiry.* Department of Health and Social Security, London.

Ham, C. (1986) *Health Policy in Britain.* Macmillan, London.

Harvey, G. (1998) Improving patient care: getting to grips with clinical governance. *RCN Magazine*, Autumn.

HMSO (2002) *The Local Authority (Overview and Scrutiny Committees Health Scrutiny Functions) Regulations 2002.* Statutory Instrument 2002 No. 3048. http://www.opsi.gov.uk/si/si2002/20023048.htm.

HMSO (2003) *Health and Social Care (Community Health and Standards) Act 2003.* Chapter 43. www.opsi.gov.uk/acts/acts2003/30043--d.htm.

Jarrold, K. (2005) Being a better manager. *Health Service Journal*, 8 December, p. 35.

King's Fund (1999) *Briefing; What Is Clinical Governance?* King's Fund, London.

The Lancet (1998) Editorial: first lessons from the 'Bristol case'. *The Lancet*, 351 (9117) 1669.

McNeil, J. (1998) Clinical governance: the whys, whats, and hows for theatre practitioners. *British Journal of Theatre Nursing*, 9 (5) 208–216.

McSherry, R. (1996) Multidisciplinary approach to patient communication. *Nursing Times*, 92 (8) 42–43.

McSherry, R. (1999) Supporting patients and their families. In: Bassett, C.C. & Makin, L. *Caring for the Seriously Ill Patient.* Arnold, London.

McSherry, R. (2004) Practice development and health care governance: a recipe for modernisation. *Journal of Nursing Management*, (12) 137–146.

McSherry, R. & Haddock, J. (1999) Evidence based health care: its place within clinical governance. *British Journal of Nursing*, 8 (2) 113–117.

McSherry, R. and Johnson, S. (eds) (2005) *Demystifying the Nurse/Therapist Consultant. A Foundation Text.* Nelson Thornes Ltd, Cheltenham.

National Statistics (2004) *Life Expectancy: More Aged 70 and 80 Than Ever Before.* www.statistics.gov.uk/cci/nugget.asp?id=881.

Press Association (2005) Obesity levels continue to rise. *The Guardian*, 16 December.

Scally, G. & Donaldson, L.J. (1998) Clinical governance and the drive for quality improvement in the new NHS in England. *BMJ*, 317, 61–65.

Stroke Unit Trialists' Collaboration (1998) Organised inpatient (stroke unit) care after stroke. In: *Stroke Module of the Cochrane Database of Systematic Reviews* (C. Warlow, J. Van Gijn & P. Sandercock, eds). BMJ Publishing Group, London.

Swage, T. (1998) Clinical care takes center stage. *Nursing Times*, 94 (14) 40–41.

The Bristol Royal Infirmary Inquiry (2001) *The Report of the Public Enquiry into Children's Heart Surgery at the Bristol Royal Infirmary 1984–1995: Learning from Bristol.* CM 5207 (I). HMSO, London. http://www.bristol-inquiry.org.uk/final_report/index.htm.

The Shipman Inquiry (2005) *The Shipman Inquiry.* http://www.the-shipman-inquiry.org.uk/finalreport.asp. HMSO, London.

Wilson, J. & Tingle, J. (1999) *Clinical Risk Modification: A Route to Clinical Governance.* Butterworth Heinemann, Oxford.

Chapter 2

What Is Clinical Governance?

Rob McSherry and Paddy Pearce

Introduction

In Chapter 1 the contributing factors that led to the introduction of clinical governance were described and discussed. This chapter explores and explains where clinical governance originated, how this concept was introduced into the NHS and its implications for healthcare professionals, managers, Trust boards and organisations.

The evolution of clinical governance

The term clinical governance can be traced to the White Paper *The New NHS: Modern, Dependable* (DH 1997). This document outlines the New Labour government's strategy for the modernisation of the NHS, with clinical governance described as:

> 'a system which is able to demonstrate, in both primary and secondary care, that systems are in place guaranteeing clinical quality improvements at all levels of healthcare provision. Healthcare organisations will be accountable for the quality of the services they provide.' (McSherry & Haddock 1999, p. 113)

In essence, clinical governance, in the authors' opinion, is viewed as the panacea for the NHS, which is perceived to be failing (as reported in the media). Prior to describing what the authors believe and understand to mean by the term clinical governance, a fundamental question requires answering. Where did clinical governance stem from?

Origins of clinical governance

Clinical governance evolved out of the term corporate governance, which originated primarily from the business world associated with the London

Stock Exchange. The intention of corporate governance in this instance was to safeguard shareholders' investments and companies' assets, the principle being that of protecting investors and minimising company risks from fraud and malpractice, e.g. the demise of Barings Bank as a result of the practices of Nick Leeson (Friedman 1995). In an attempt to prevent similar incidents within the UK stock exchange, the Cadbury Committee was established. In 1992 this committee defined corporate governance as 'the system by which companies are directed and controlled' (NHS Executive 1999).

The Cadbury Committee identified three fundamental requirements to assure corporate governance within organisations:

- Internal financial controls, i.e. the annual auditing of financial accounts to ensure appropriate use of the company's finances without any underhand dealings.
- Efficient and effective operations, i.e. the company is providing value for money.
- Compliance with laws and regulations, i.e. health and safety is not being compromised; employers and the public are protected.

This was termed the 'Cadbury Code'. This code was enhanced by the Greenbury and Hemple Committees, resulting in the publication by the London Stock Exchange of a Combined Code of Principles of Good Governance.

The code's major recommendations were that 'the board should maintain a sound system of internal control to safeguard shareholders' investments and company assets . . . The directors should, at least annually, conduct a review of the effectiveness of the group's systems of internal control and should report to the shareholders that they have done so. The review should cover all controls, including financial, operational, and compliance controls and risk management.' (NHS Executive 1999)

Basically this means that corporate governance is about having a systematic approach to demonstrate that the company is doing its best to protect investors' monies and the company's future, and is complying with statutory obligations. To achieve this, all the company's operational processes require regular monitoring and reviewing in an open and transparent manner.

The Cadbury Code was improved by the Turnbull Committee, which reported in 1999, recommending the need for adequately resourced internal audit departments to evaluate risk and monitor the effectiveness of the company's performance. The potential benefits from corporate governance in the independent sector – open channels of communication, safeguarding public and employees, and demonstrating value for money – could equally be applied to the public sector. The government, in an attempt to demonstrate its commitment to improving public service provision, embraced the standards of corporate governance by introducing the principles of corporate governance into the NHS in 1994.

Corporate governance and the NHS

Activity 2.1

How do you think the principles of corporate governance may apply to the NHS?

Read on and then compare your responses with those in the feedback box at the end of this section.

Corporate governance was introduced into the NHS via a three-stage process, which is continuing. This process is described below.

The development of a framework of corporate governance

This was outlined in the publication *Corporate Governance in the NHS; Code of Conduct and Code of Accountability* (NHS Executive 1999), where the focus of the document was directed at NHS Trust boards in order to ensure and demonstrate that the conduct of the board was exemplary. The code of conduct for NHS boards is based on three principles as shown in Box 2.1.

Box 2.1   Principles of corporate governance in the NHS (DH 1994)

- **Accountability** – everything done by those who work in the NHS must be able to stand the test of parliamentary scrutiny, public judgements on propriety and professional codes of conduct.
- **Probity** – there should be an absolute standard of honesty in dealing with the assets of the NHS: integrity should be the hallmark of all personal conduct in decisions affecting patients, staff and suppliers, and in the use of information acquired in the course of NHS duties.
- **Openness** – there should be sufficient transparency about NHS activities to promote confidence between the NHS authority or Trust and its staff, patients and the public.

Essentially the code of conduct and accountability is about ensuring that each member of staff knows who he or she is accountable to and for what practices. This should occur in an honest and open environment. Basically this means telling the truth when things go right and when things go wrong.

Improvements in the organisation and staffing of internal audit

This is about ensuring that internal systems are in place throughout the organisation that are working well in highlighting good practice and areas in need of improvement; for example, periodic auditing of staff expenses claims, and vetting the tendering process where external contractors are bidding for NHS work, to gain the best possible quote and ensure value for money.

The development of controls assurance

Controls assurance can be viewed as part of governance and is described as 'a holistic concept based on best governance practice' (NHS Executive 1999, p. 2); that means meeting the codes of conduct and accountability as previously mentioned. Controls assurance is concerned with methods that enable healthcare organisations to provide evidence that they are doing their 'reasonable best' to manage risk and demonstrate to the public and all stakeholders that they are doing so. Controls assurance is described in more detail later in this chapter.

In summary, corporate governance within the NHS is concerned with the non-clinical aspects of healthcare provision that are ensuring financial and operational success by demonstrating value for money. The link to achieve total governance is that of combining the non-clinical with the clinical aspects of healthcare provision. Perhaps this is the primary influence that resulted in the government's introduction of 'clinical governance' within the NHS.

Activity 2.1: Feedback

Corporate governance is about protecting investors' monies and companies' assets from risks. If these principles are paralleled to the NHS, then corporate governance is about having efficient and effective systems in place to show that money is not being wasted and the services are providing value for money. This is because the NHS is publicly funded via taxation, placing a moral and statutory duty on the management and employees to demonstrate how and where that public money is being spent.

As employees, whether in public or independent sectors, we are governed by contracts of employment, professional regulations and ultimately the civil and criminal laws to provide the best possible service within the given resources. The key word that springs to mind in ensuring corporate governance is accountability. Accountability means that you are able to justify your actions – essentially what you do and why you have to do it.

Defining clinical governance

This section outlines the original definition of clinical governance and then reviews the working definitions provided by some of the healthcare disciplines. The review compares and contrasts existing definitions, culminating in a practical definition by the authors, along with identification of the key themes of clinical governance, which are expanded upon in Chapter 3.

As mentioned above, the term clinical governance can be traced to the New Labour government's first White Paper on health, *The New NHS: Modern, Dependable* (DH 1997). This sets out the government's aims of making the NHS modern and dependable, by keeping what has worked in the past and discarding what has failed; for example, by abolishing the internal market that placed finance and activity above clinical quality, leading to fragmentation of services and the ideology of command and control. To resolve these failings the government's philosophy is that of partnerships and collaboration, where innovation is nurtured and staff are valued. The latter is to be achieved by the application of six key principles (see Box 2.2).

Box 2.2   The principles of clinical governance

1. To re-establish the NHS as a national service for all patients throughout the country, where patients will receive high quality care regardless of age, gender or culture if they are ill or injured.
2. To establish national standards based upon best practices, which will be influenced and delivered locally by the healthcare professionals themselves, taking into account the needs of the local population.
3. Collaborative working partnerships between hospitals, community services and local authorities, where the patient is the central focus.
4. To ensure that the healthcare services are delivering high quality care and providing value for money.
5. To establish an internal culture where clinical quality is guaranteed for all patients.
6. To enhance public confidence in the NHS.

Adapted from DH (1997)

The new structures and systems proposed to achieve the six key principles were laid out in a set of national service frameworks (NSFs) to be developed with nationally agreed standards. These covered major care areas and disease groups, e.g. cancer services, heart disease, mental health and caring for the older person. The purpose of the NSFs is to provide sound, equitable and consistent evidence-based care and services (DH 2000a, p. 7). Today there are nine NSFs, covering the areas of mental health, coronary heart disease, diabetes, renal care, older people, children, cancer, paediatric intensive care and long-term conditions.

The National Institute for Clinical Excellence (NICE) is responsible for the assessment of new technologies and producing robust and authoritative guidelines for the NHS. In 2004, a newly established organisation – the Commission for Healthcare Audit and Inspection – took over from the Commission for Health Improvement (CHI). This organisation is commonly referred to as the Healthcare Commission (HC). The purpose of this organisation is to monitor the quality of clinical services at a local level, intervene if necessary, deal with problems and provide parliament with an annual report on the state of the NHS. Furthermore, the HC is responsible for monitoring the overall performance of the NHS against *Standards for Better Health* (DH 2004). These are discussed later in the chapter.

A new performance framework with a scorecard of quality effectiveness and efficiency measures, rather than the previous cost and activity focus, has been developed. This approach to performance management has added an important dimension – ensuring that clinical care and patient outcome is given equal status to that of finance, cost and activity. The approach has led to the development of the HC Annual Health Check, which adopts an even broader view to performance management for the NHS. Performance management is discussed in more detail in Chapter 3.

The new system of clinical governance is able to demonstrate, in both primary and secondary care, that systems are in place guaranteeing clinical quality improvements at all levels of healthcare provision.

The structures identified above are all individually directed towards establishing and monitoring the level of clinical quality at individual, organisational, regional and national levels; for example, NICE will set standards and guidelines based on the best available evidence accessible nationally for use by individual health professionals. The role of local NHS and Primary Care Trusts together with Strategic Health Authorities will be to implement these guidelines. The CHI and subsequently the HC has the role of monitoring healthcare organisations to ensure that these standards are achieved.

Clinical governance, according to Donaldson (1998), is viewed as the vehicle to achieve, locally, continuous improvements in clinical quality, which will aid the government's agenda for modernisation of the NHS, evident from the following statement:

'Chief executives will be expected to ensure there are appropriate local arrangements to give them and the NHS Trust board firm assurances that their responsibilities for quality are being met. This might be through the creation of a Board Sub Committee, led by a named senior consultant, nurse, or other clinical professional, with responsibility for ensuring the internal clinical governance of the organisation.' (DH 1997, p. 47)

A considerable amount of literature is emerging on the topic of clinical governance, regarding what it is and what it is perceived to be within the various healthcare professions (see Table. 2.1). According to this table, the government's initial definition of clinical governance seems to have been embraced by the majority of healthcare professions. However, some differences emerge in the way individual professions have interpreted, internalised and transferred the meaning of clinical governance to their specific profession. For instance, occupational therapy views clinical governance 'as a framework for combining a full range of quality activities, building first upon what is already being carried out' (Sealey 1999). This definition by Sealey (1999) infers that it is essential to build on existing good practice in a systematic and organised manner. Similarly the Royal College of Nursing (RCN) (1998) defines clinical governance as 'a framework, which helps all clinicians including nurses to continuously improve quality and safeguard standards of care'. The RCN (1998), like Sealey (1999), considers clinical governance as a framework for maintaining, sustaining and improving standards but differs in the way it acknowledges the importance of clinical governance to all professional groups. Omission of these definitions along with the others provided is a failure to capture the multi- and inter-professional relevance of clinical governance, for example the contributions from the many other groups such as clerical, administration, finance, human resources, ancillary, maintenance and engineering staff.

There are a number of common emergent themes from the definitions offered by the various professional groups, with the majority viewing clinical governance as a Department of Health directive through which individuals and organisations are accountable for clinical quality, service and patient safety. Most definitions acknowledge the fact that clinical governance is a framework that pulls a whole range of organisational departments together by focusing on the systems and processes, with a strong emphasis placed on accountability associated with the maintenance and improvement of standards. Clinical governance for us draws together a number of concepts; namely:

- The systematic harmonisation of clinical and managerial responsibilities with accountable practice
- Team working and interdependency
- Monitoring, changing, evaluating and improving practice to safeguard standards
- The drive for constant quality improvement in all that we do
- Nurturing a culture of continuous learning
- Placing a duty of care to improve individual, team and organisational performance.

Table 2.1 A critical review of professional perspectives in defining clinical governance.

Author	Year	Professional discipline	Definition	Key themes
Department of Health	1997	Government	'A framework through which NHS organizations are accountable for continuously improving the quality of their services and safeguarding high standards of care by creating an environment in which excellence in clinical care will flourish'	Framework Accountability Maintaining Improvement Culture Quality Prospering
Sealey	1999	Occupational therapists	'A framework for combining a full range of quality activities, building first upon what is already being carried out'	Framework Quality Maintaining Improvement
McNeil	1998	Theatre nurses	'The means by which organizations ensure the provision of quality clinical care by making individuals accountable for setting, maintaining and monitoring performance standards'	Quality Accountability Maintaining Improving Standards Outcome

Table 2.1   *(cont'd)*

Author	Year	Professional discipline	Definition	Key themes
Scally & Donaldson	1998	Doctors	'The main vehicle for continuously improving the quality of patient care and developing the capacity of the NHS in England to maintain high standards'	Quality Improvement Maintaining Resource Standards
Royal College of General Practitioners	2005	GPs	'The principal aims of clinical governance are to improve the quality and the accountability of healthcare'	Improvement Quality Accountability
Royal College of Nursing	1998	Nurses	'A framework which helps all clinicians – including nurses – to continuously improve quality and safeguard standards of care'	Framework Improvement Maintaining Quality Standards Indirectly accountability

European Region of the World Confederation for Physical Therapy	2003	Physiotherapists	'A government initiative (introduced in 1998) to provide a framework through which NHS organisations are accountable for continuously improving the quality of services they deliver'	Framework Accountability Quality Improvement
British Dental Association	2006	Dentists	'Is part of the NHS drive to improve the quality of health care and to make providers accountable for delivering a consistent standard on which patients can rely'	Improvement Quality Accountability Delivery Standards
Royal Pharmaceutical Society of Great Britain	2005	Pharmacists	'The means by which organisations ensure the provision of quality clinical care by making individuals accountable for setting, maintaining and monitoring standards'	Quality Accountability Maintaining Monitoring Standards
Association of Optometrists	2003	Optometrists	'Has to do with the delivery of high quality clinical services. Clinical governance is to be a welcomed as it makes clinical quality an integral part of the NHS governance framework'	Delivery Quality Framework

The prominent theme from the various definitions is the emphasis on having robust systems/frameworks for ensuring that clinical quality exists throughout the entire organisation, where each individual is accountable for his or her actions. We would argue that clinical governance could at best be summarised as a robust framework that acknowledges the importance of adopting a culture of shared accountability for sustaining and improving the quality of services and outcomes for both patients and staff. Clinical governance is ultimately 'an umbrella term' for all the issues and concepts that clinicians, non clinicians, mangers and board members know and foster, including standard setting, risk management, performance management, clinical audit, training, reflection and professional development to name but a few (McSherry & Haddock 1999). Clinical governance is about instilling confidence in both the public and healthcare professionals by providing them with a safe clinical environment in which to accommodate the challenges identified in Chapter 1 which are facing them in the future. In a simple way, clinical governance is about the patients/carers receiving the right care at the right time from the right person, in a safe, honest, open and caring environment. To ensure that clinical governance is successfully implemented throughout any healthcare organisation the key components contained within its definition need to be available and achievable throughout the organisation, as the following section will now briefly explain.

The key components of clinical governance

This section introduces the key components of clinical governance and how they relate to individuals, organisations and the wider aspect of the NHS; a more detailed account is offered in Chapter 3.

The definitions of clinical governance provided and identified in Table 2.1 highlight common themes that describe what clinical governance is. These can be summarised as shown in Fig. 2.1. Figure 2.1 depicts the key components that make up clinical governance, which in turn could be considered as the building blocks for its success for either an individual or a healthcare organisation. For clinical governance to operate effectively the identified components need to be evident and operational. Clinical quality and continuous improvements in healthcare delivery can only be achieved in a culture and environment that supports, values and develops its staff. Likewise, individual healthcare professionals need to continuously develop their professional standards whilst operating within the roles and responsibilities aligned to their contract of employment and codes of professional practice. Essentially clinical governance is about providing good clinical care in an environment that places patient and staff safety as a number one priority.

Fig. 2.1 Key components of clinical governance.

It is evident from the above description of the authors' interpretations of the various definitions of clinical governance identified in Table 2.1 that their primary focus is on improving the quality and standards of clinical practice, although within these definitions of clinical governance there appear to be no explicit links to the non-clinical aspects of healthcare, which are equally important in improving clinical quality.

Non-clinical services that support clinical governance

Activity 2.2: Non-clinical services that support clinical governance

List the non-clinical services that support healthcare professionals in executing clinical governance successfully.

Read on and compare your findings with those in the feedback box towards the end of the chapter.

When providing care in a busy and stressful clinical setting it is easy to forget all those other supporting services that are perhaps taken for granted when we provide our services. For example, consider the simple case of a general practitioner referring a patient to a consultant for a clinical opinion. This involves the letter from the GP, perhaps dictated for his or her clerical staff to process, which may be received by the medical records staff or consultant secretaries, who in turn arrange an outpatient appointment and inform the patient. The patient subsequently attends the outpatient department to be seen by the consultant. For this to happen effectively, much work is done behind the scenes that involves the following groups of personnel: estate staffs in maintaining the safety of the building and mains services; domestics in maintaining the cleanliness and hygiene standards; and a range of supporting services to enable the operational and clinical staff to perform their duties, such as personnel, finance and information services. Thus clinical governance cannot be operationalised without the non-clinical supporting services, as depicted by the simple example above. This example demonstrates the links between non-clinical supporting activity and clinical governance. Clinical governance cannot be successfully implemented without the support of the non-clinical aspects of healthcare delivery. As most health professionals are fully aware, healthcare provision and delivery is complex in nature. Successful healthcare delivery is dependent on good teamwork, effective leadership and sound management in drawing together the non-clinical and clinical aspects of governance. Basically neither can work effectively without the other, as outlined in Fig. 2.2.

Figure 2.2 highlights the role of healthcare governance in uniting the three elements of health service governance: corporate (management), clinical (clinical practice) and the non-clinical supporting services. Whilst

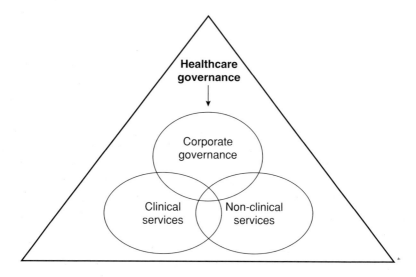

Fig. 2.2   Healthcare governance in the NHS.

there has been much attention directed towards establishing good managerial and clinical practices based on sound evidence in order to ensure clinical quality, it would appear that ensuring quality associated with the non-clinical supporting services, such as those outlined in Activity 2.2, was not given equal status. To address this imbalance it is important to know that the government initially introduced guidelines and standards for the NHS to assure quality in these parts of the organisation. This was facilitated and achieved through the introduction of 'controls assurance' (NHS Executive 1999).

Controls assurance

The Health Service Circular 1999/123 describes controls assurance as 'A holistic concept based on best governance practice' (NHS Executive 1999, p. 2). This approach is reinforced and enhanced by Emslie, who defines controls assurance as:

> 'a process, built on best governance practice, by which NHS organisations demonstrate that they are doing their reasonable best to manage themselves so as to meet their objectives and protect patients, staff, visitors, and other stakeholders against risks of all kinds.' (Emslie 2001, p. 1)

The difficulty for many healthcare organisations and individuals is in conceptualising and implementing healthcare governance, because they see each component, such as clinical governance, corporate governance and controls assurance, as separate and unrelated entities. The authors accept that many healthcare professionals view the components of healthcare governance in isolation, but we would argue that in practice this is usually not the case. For example, the routine administration of either an intravenous or an intramuscular injection involves many clinical and non-clinical healthcare professionals and systems and processes in order to work efficiently and effectively. Some healthcare professionals only see their part of the overall systems and process(es), such as the preparation and administration. However, what happens if the medication and equipment are not available or the 'sharps' are not disposed of safely? This simple illustration demonstrates that healthcare governance is truly a holistic concept that unifies the three components of clinical, non-clinical and corporate governance. Controls assurance is the vehicle that enables each organisation to demonstrate that its systems and processes for assuring healthcare governance are both efficient and effective.

Emslie (2001) provides a model linking corporate (Trust) objectives with providing assurance to stakeholders of quality healthcare, highlighting the importance of accountability, processes, capability and outcomes, of which each element is continuously monitored and reviewed, and where lessons are learnt, practices improved and risks minimised. Essentially this model can be applied to individuals, teams and organisations. Controls assurance was concerned with methods that enable healthcare organisations to provide evidence that they are doing their 'reasonable best' to manage risk and demonstrate to the public and all stakeholders that they are doing so. The main principle underpinning controls assurance is that of collaborative working, thus ensuring that risks are minimised and where identified are managed appropriately (McSherry & Pearce 2000; Emslie 2001).

Within the Health Service Circular HSC 1999/123, chief executives were advised to appoint an executive director to assume responsibility for the implementation of controls assurance, thus making an individual the accountable officer to parliament. The designated person was charged with reviewing the circular and guidance. Chief executives were responsible for informing the National Controls Assurance Project Manager, who is the designated person for their organisation.

The HSC 1999/123 led to the development of 18 standards covering the non-clinical and some clinical aspects of service delivery, such as infection control, health and safety and waste management. The standards were released on 22 November 1999 at the NHS Controls Assurance Conference, forming 'the basis of a self-assessment exercise to be undertaken by all NHS trusts and health authorities from 2000, leading up to an assurance statement to be signed by chief executives on behalf of boards in their 1999–2000 annual report' (Hopkins 2000, p. 22). In essence, controls assurance completed the governance picture by linking the corporate, clinical and non-clinical elements of governance.

More information on controls assurance can be found by reading McSherry and Pearce (2000), NHS Executive (1999) and Hopkins (2000). It is clear from Fig. 2.1 that the key elements of governance all have potential benefits to improve the quality of care, which can be further enhanced when these components work in harmony. Since the introduction of the controls assurance standards the NHS has realised the need to adopt an integrated approach to healthcare governance. As a consequence, today healthcare governance, as highlighted previously by Stanton (2004), could be viewed as a Rubik cube, incorporating the six faces of governance (Fig. 2.3).

It is evident from Fig. 2.3 that the concept of healthcare governance has evolved, incorporating additional elements to those highlighted previously in Fig 2.2. Healthcare governance has become a phrase that demonstrates the importance of adopting an integrated approach to governance in its totality. Healthcare governance today involves clinical governance, information governance, financial governance, controls

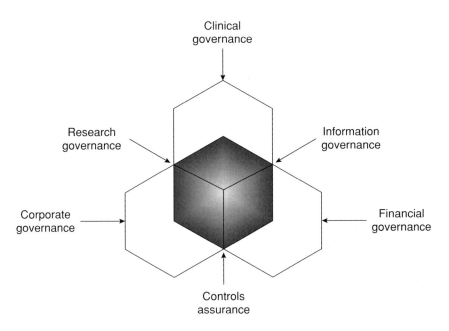

Fig. 2.3   The six faces of healthcare governance.

assurance, corporate governance and research governance. Like the Rubik cube, the benefits can only be fully realised when the six faces of each cube are aligned. Put simply, integrated or healthcare governance is dependent on the efficient and effective alignment and co-ordination of the various components of governance. Similarly, at an organisational level the various departments that constitute the six faces of the Rubik cube need to co-operate and communicate effectively in an open culture of mutual respect and co-operation. As a consequence of adopting this whole systems approach to governance we have witnessed the demise of controls assurance standards (Pearce 2004) for the NHS organisation, being replaced by the Standards for Better Health (DH 2004). These are discussed in the next section.

Standards for Better Health

The section is reproduced from the Healthcare Risk Report with kind permission of Lexis Nexis. The information is based upon the work of McSherry and Pearce (2004) entitled 'Healthcare Standards: A Critique of the Department of Health's National Standards for the NHS'.

The introduction of the DH's Standards for Better Health (DH 2004) can be attributed to a combination of several issues involving societal, political and professional factors. These include changes in health policy, influenced by the Prime Minister's principles surrounding public sector reform, rising patient/carer expectations, increased patient dependency, technology advances, demographic changes in society, changes in care delivery systems, lack of public confidence in the NHS, threat of litigation and demand for greater access to information (McSherry & McSherry 2001).

Activity 2.3

What do you understand by the term national healthcare standards? Why do you think these have been developed? What aspects of healthcare do you think these standards should cover?

Read on and then compare your responses with those in the feedback box at the end of this section.

The need for national healthcare standards

The provision of accessible, equitable, high-quality care and services is difficult for the NHS to achieve. The ideal is a service that provides high-quality services delivered locally by well-trained, motivated people, that delivers the right care to the right individual in the right setting at the right time (McSherry & Pearce 2002). This approach to service provision must be capable of demonstrating success in a meaningful way to patients, the public, healthcare organisations and ultimately the government.

As highlighted in the previous chapter, in recent years a number of major clinical and corporate failures in the NHS have attracted adverse media coverage (Smith 1998). The Bristol Royal Infirmary Inquiry found the outcomes and care of children undergoing cardiac surgery there to be suboptimal, while the Royal Liverpool Children's Inquiry found that at Alder Hey Children's Hospital, body parts of children were removed and kept without the informed consent of parents. The public and government have realised that the NHS was not delivering what the public expected, including clinical outcomes comparable with other western nations. So, what has happened to address service failures and indeed to fulfil the founding aspirational principles of the NHS?

The concept of performance management (detailed in Chapter 3) has been introduced and over the decades the NHS has been subjected to an ever-increasing number of targets and performance measures. A reductionist approach is evident and often what is measured is that which can be counted, such as waiting times in accident and emergency. We would suggest that this approach has been extended to the concept of 'inspection', in this instance referring to internal and external inspection and review to assure the government and the public that the NHS is delivering good quality outcomes.

NHS organisations are reviewed by a diverse range of inspectorates covering a broad spectrum of NHS activity. These inspecting organisations appear to work in splendid isolation, often examining similar areas from a slightly different perspective and on occasion reaching very different conclusions. These inconsistencies lead to confusion over the expectations of the inspectorates, placing ever-increasing demands on NHS organisations, which deploy disproportionate resources to achieve targets and prepare for inspection. The present government's NHS Plan (DH 2000b) promises investment and reform through modernisation. The NHS has undoubtedly been subjected to over-inspection, with the emphasis on targets leading to low morale and demotivated staff. This point was highlighted in the Bristol Royal Infirmary Inquiry report and the recommendation was made that 'the NHS should have national standards'. In response the DH has attempted to produce national generic standards for the entire service.

Defining the healthcare standards

Healthcare standards in the Bristol report are being defined as a level, which others accept as the baseline for good practice, or the desired level of achievement (Schroeder & Maibusch 1984). Successive DH White Papers (DH 1997, 1998) have placed emphasis on the importance of improving and assuring quality of care, treatment and services through the principles of clinical governance. This is a major feature in guaranteeing quality to the public and ensuring that clinical, managerial and educational practice within the NHS are based on measurable evidence (McSherry & Haddock 1999). Quality improvements have been placed at the forefront of the NHS agenda and clinical effectiveness is to be measured and evaluated against the proposed set of healthcare standards.

We would argue that there is a definite need for an integrated approach to the establishment of healthcare standards in the NHS. Organisational standards and accreditation schemes are essential for demonstrating acquired levels of excellence within any organisation. They provide excellent frameworks for promoting quality improvements, and as a result support organisations and professionals in making practice open and accountable. Our recent experiences of working with organisational standards, along with assessing levels of achieved practice, identify that they require organisational and managerial support, resources and financial backing.

Organisational standard measurement is an integral part of quality improvement. Practice areas need to provide evidence to the accrediting bodies to show how they have achieved a particular standard. Bodies such as the Healthcare Commission and the National Health Service Litigation Authority (NHSLA) through its Clinical Negligence Scheme for Trusts require practice areas to demonstrate how they are providing effective quality care. The difficulties and challenges in the development of healthcare standards are in producing criteria against which they can be easily, consistently and uniformly assessed, which is perhaps a limitation for some existing healthcare standards and accrediting bodies. The way forward to resolving these and many other issues aligned to healthcare standards and accreditation is the production of a generic framework. The government is at least trying to address these issues by consulting with organisations and users of healthcare services on the proposed healthcare standards.

Describing the new healthcare standards

The document *Standards for Better Health: Healthcare Standards for Services Under the NHS – A Consultation* (DH 2004) was published in February 2004 for a three-month consultation period. The then Secretary of State John Reid states in the foreword:

> 'These standards are not yet another batch of rules and regulations whose object is to tie clinicians into further procedures and targets.' (DH 2004, p. 2)

The document has six key sections, of which section three details 24 core standards and section four outlines ten developmental standards. These two sections are the key sections with which healthcare organisations and professionals should become familiar. The core standards attempt to set out clearly what patients can expect from the NHS. They do not seek to establish new standards but bring together the vast array of complex and confusing guidelines, measures and assessments. In contrast, developmental standards are not absolute measures, but more broad-based, concerned with assessing progress made with implementation of the NHS Plan and other key NHS strategy documents. The challenge for the organisation is in ensuring that it implements and reviews the core standards alongside the developmental standards. The 24 four core standards are set out within seven domains (see Box 2.3).

According to Box 2.3 it would appear that the DH is attempting to provide an integrated approach towards governance. The similarities of the domains with the clinical and corporate governance framework are strik-

---

Box 2.3 The seven domains of healthcare standards

- Safety
- Clinical and cost effectiveness
- Governance
- Patient focus
- Accessible and responsive care
- Care environment and amenities
- Public health

---

ing (McSherry & Pearce 2002). However, what is behind each of these domains needs further exploration.

Safety is defined as 'the design of health care processes, working practices and systematic activities to prevent or reduce risk of harm to patients'. There are five associated standards predominantly centred on risk, risk management and learning from experience good and not so good. One standard is a developmental standard, concerning the introduction and enhancement of the systems and processes to monitor and respond to risks continuously.

The definition of clinical and cost effectiveness is that 'health care decisions are based on what appropriately assessed research evidence has shown provides an effective outcome for patients' individual needs'. There are two core standards and one developmental standard. The emphasis is on ensuring that care and treatments are based on best available evidence and guidance.

The definition of governance is that 'all providers of health services have in place the managerial and clinical leadership and accountability, the organisational culture, and the systems and working practices to enable probity, quality assurance, quality improvement and patient safety to be central components of all routines, processes and activities'. This domain is the most comprehensive standard and includes seven core standards and three developmental standards. The emphasis is on integration of clinical and corporate governance frameworks into a holistic and integrated governance model.

Patient focus is defined as healthcare that 'is provided in partnership with patients, their carers and relatives and is designed around decisions which respect their diverse needs, preferences and choices'. The domain includes four core standards and two developmental standards. The central aims of these standards are ensuring equity, equal access to information, the maintenance of confidentiality, and the involvement of carers and patients in their care and treatment and the design/development of new services. By extension we would argue that all of the NHS must be patient-focused.

Accessible and responsive care is identified as patients receiving services as promptly as possible, having choice in access to services and treatments, and experiencing the minimum unnecessary delay at any stage of service delivery or the care pathway. The domain contains two core standards and one developmental standard, reinforcing the need for healthcare organisations and services to focus their attention on ensuring access and equity of services. It is notable that the patient focus and accessible and responsive care domains go hand in hand and could easily be incorporated as one domain.

Care environment and amenities identifies that care should be 'provided in environments that promote patient and staff well-being and respect for patients' needs and preferences, in that they are designed for the effective and safe delivery of treatment, care or a specific function (such as catering or pharmacy), accord an appropriate degree of privacy, are well maintained and are cleaned to optimise health outcomes'. This domain includes one core standard and one developmental standard, emphasising the need for organisations and individuals to actively consider safety, support, patient privacy and confidentiality. It could be argued that traditionally environmental factors have not been seen as a high priority, yet they are fundamental to patient and staff well-being.

Public health is a new area for standard-setting in the NHS. Public health in this instance is defined as providing 'leadership, and collaborat[ing] with relevant local organisations and communities to ensure the design and delivery of programmes and services which promote, protect and improve the health of the population and reduce inequalities between different population groups and areas'. This is a highly topical and important domain because of changes in demography and society. Furthermore this is an underdeveloped field of practice for many healthcare professionals to implement. The success of this domain depends on developing partnerships and co-operative strategies with other public and commercial enterprises. Primary care trusts should drive this domain forward.

The standards vs existing systems

There are several pros and cons that seem to surround the introduction of national healthcare standards for the NHS. The concept of a set of national standards that try to draw together the key components of the business of the NHS is essential, given the disparity and inequity of service that continues to exist within the NHS. NHS organisations and professionals welcome the introduction of a set of national standards, providing they support professional practice and quality improvement and do not add further to the bureaucracy of existing systems of performance review. However, as the NHS is such a complex and multifaceted organisation, is it really possible to introduce such a framework? Previous attempts have resulted in crude measures, such as the NHS performance indicators, and have led to a lack of confidence in the systems because they were meant to be supportive, proactive and not reactive and policing (McSherry & Pearce 2002).

The greatest weakness of this document in our minds is that the DH has written the standards and the Healthcare Commission has been asked to provide criteria to measure compliance. There is a suggestion that the Commission will try to use what currently exists. However, we would argue that the vision of the Commission is to reduce the burden of inspection on the NHS, and not to make it even more complex and demanding. To adopt this approach will require genuine collaboration between those operating schemes such as Investors in People (IIP), the Clinical Negligence Scheme for Trusts (CNST) and controls assurance. Is this really possible?

Some years ago, the CHI, NHSLA and others formed the NHS Reviews Coordination Group, which in 2002 produced a document called *Principles of Agreement*, aiming to improve the efficiency of reviews of risk management. Yet each organisation continues to disregard the findings of each other and continues to examine common areas and issues from slightly different perspectives. The NHSLA has produced a CNST risk management standard for primary care trusts, similar to the core risk management standard of the annual controls assurance standards assessment that all NHS bodies must undertake. Could it be argued that the healthcare standards are a duplication of the above or could the healthcare standards endorse the existing standards within these standards as a form of external assurance?

The challenge for some NHS organisations will be in applying these healthcare standards to existing practice, and marrying existing standards of accreditation within the healthcare standards. This has been particularly challenging for PCTs with regard to commissioned services and independent contractors. Furthermore, will the Healthcare Commission be able to devise a robust set of criteria to assess these standards in order to measure essential developmental aspects of a service?

Applying the healthcare standards to an example of practice

For the healthcare standards to become an integral part of demonstrable healthcare quality and improvement it is fundamental they become adopted by and applied at all levels of the NHS. To this end a whole systems approach to healthcare governance needs to be developed (McSherry 2004). Figure 2.4 attempts to show how the seven domains of the healthcare

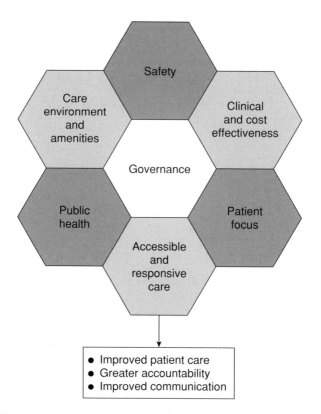

Fig. 2.4   The interdependent relationship of healthcare standards.

standards fit together and that they are interdependent on each other through the use of a whole systems approach to quality improvement.

This approach recognises the need for an integrated approach to healthcare governance, where through the development of interdependent relationships it is more likely to succeed. It can be applied to all NHS organisations as it represents the very core of our business, delivering high-quality patient-focused care locally. We would argue that this encourages clinical and non-clinical staff to harmonise efforts for the good and benefit of patients in a coordinated and efficient manner.

The new healthcare standards highlighted in Fig. 2.4 will only be effective through the adoption of a whole systems approach. A whole systems approach reinforces the concept of healthcare governance applicable at an organisational and individual level, and shows how the essential components of each concept can be applied and reviewed under the key domains of safety, clinical and cost effectiveness, governance, patient focus, accessible and responsive care, care environment and amenities and public health. Whilst the above framework is associated with competency or performance-related issues at an organisational, department/directorate and team level, the same could be used for promoting the NHS modernisation agenda. The key to successful modernisation through the healthcare standards is associated with harmonising (or integration) of the clinical and non-clinical aspects of governance, as described in the following section.

Criteria for evaluating the standards

For successful implementation of the healthcare standards it is imperative that the Healthcare Commission uses its authority to encourage all inspectorates to unite. Unification of these various organisational accrediting bodies is imperative. The key disadvantage of organisational standards and accreditation within the NHS today is in the duplication of time, resources and support needed for individuals, teams and organisations in collecting, collating and providing evidence. Health and social care organisations seem to be pressurised in meeting the criteria not just for one award but for several at any one time (Kell *et al.* 2004).

A critical review of the organisational and accreditation frameworks such as IIP, the European Foundation for Quality Management (EFQM), CNST and Charter Mark has already revealed a set of the primary core themes in the publication of the Excellence in Practice Accreditation Scheme (EPAS) (McSherry *et al.* 2003). EPAS provides a robust framework supporting the clinical governance agenda because of its associations with the key components of clinical governance. There are many examples of organisational accreditation schemes, but none of them captures the essence of clinical governance or evidence-based practice within a practice development framework. The uniqueness of the EPAS is in collectively addressing the key issues in developing, advancing and evaluating practice, which could easily be transferred and further developed to incorporate the non-clinical aspects of the integrated governance model and healthcare standards.

The acid test for the healthcare standards and ultimately the commission itself will be in demonstrating a reduction in the burden of inspection, by the use of intelligent information that ultimately leads to targeted and proportionate inspection. The Standards for Better Health have currently been in place for two years, but for the financial year 2005–2006 NHS organisations were required to make a declaration of compliance against the 24 core standards. These are considered to be the basic standards that should be currently achieved by all NHS organisations. Since the original consultation and publication of *Standards for Better Health* (DH 2004), the HC has published a consultation document on compliance with the Development Standards (HC 2005). This document indicates an increase from 10 to 13 standards, notably around safety.

Activity 2.2: Feedback: Non-clinical services that support the implementation of clinical governance

Note: this is by no means an exhaustive list and is not placed in any order of priority.

- Finance
- Personnel (human resources)
- Estates: building, electrical and mechanical services
- Catering
- Domestic services
- Information technology
- Administration and clerical services
- Medical records
- Library services

Activity 2.3: Feedback

Standards for Better Health adopt a much broader approach to performance management, taking into consideration the perspectives of the DH, health-care professionals and, more importantly, patients and carers, providing a clear set of standards that all NHS organisations should be meeting. This new approach attempts to integrate the various NHS structures and systems within an organisation using a whole systems approach.

Conclusion

In conclusion, clinical governance is a highly complex and multifaceted concept, dependent upon successful adoption of a whole systems approach that integrates the clinical and non-clinical services. The successful integration of these various elements within any healthcare organisation we believe could result in the achievement of 'healthcare governance'. Healthcare governance is about establishing frameworks for sustaining and improving clinical quality, which can only take place when the organisational infrastructures support the overall aims of corporate, clinical and non-clinical aspects of governance.

Garside (1999) reinforces our term 'healthcare governance' by suggesting that clinical governance is 'the opportunity to change systems – to pull together different components and strands from the clinical and managerial worlds to improve things for patients'. The challenge for the NHS is in 'converging' all of the governance components identified in Fig. 2.3 under a single umbrella which all healthcare professionals can access, understand, implement and evaluate at a level most suited to their roles and responsibilities in an attempt to minimise risks. Convergence has already been recognised by the DH:

> 'We are committed to achieving a fully integrated approach to governance where clinical and corporate governance sit side by side – clinical governance focusing on continuous improvements in quality and corporate governance focusing on having the necessary systems in place to minimise risk.' (Reeves 2001, p. 1)

The Health Service Circular 2001/005 (NHS Executive 2001) provides advice and guidance together with a timetable for this to occur within the NHS by 2005. In 2005 the DH introduced the term 'integrated governance' and has recently published guidance on what this means for NHS organisations (DH 2006). Yet, we believe the term tends to focus on organisational and managerial aspects of an NHS organisation at higher levels, appearing to have limited relevance and application to staff in their daily work. To develop understanding of clinical governance, the key components will be examined in detail in Chapter 3.

Key points

Corporate governance
Corporate governance in general is about protecting investors' monies and companies' assets from risks. Likewise corporate governance in the NHS is about ensuring that public monies have not been wasted in healthcare delivery.

Clinical governance
Clinical governance is a framework for the continual improvement of patient care by minimising clinical risks and continuing the development of organisations and staff.

Healthcare governance
Healthcare governance is the harmonisation of corporate governance, clinical governance and controls assurance.

Suggested reading

Hopkins, B. (2000) National Controls Assurance Conference. *Health Care Risk Report*, 6 (3) 22–24.

NHS Executive (1999) *Health Services Circular 1999/123. Governance in the New NHS: Controls Assurance Statements 1999/2000: Risk Management and Organizational Controls*. DH, London.

RCN (2000) *Clinical Governance: How Nurses Can Get Involved*. Royal College of Nursing, London.

Roland, M. & Baker, R. (1999) *Clinical Governance Practical Guide for Primary Care Teams*. The National Primary Care Research and Development Centre, University of Manchester and University of Leicester.

Smith, S. (1998) Model behaviour. *Nursing Management*, 5 (6) 19–24.

Useful websites

Department of Health Governance:
www.dh.gov.uk/PolicyAndGuidance/OrganisationPolicy/Governance/fs/en

References

Association of Optometrists (2003) *Clinical Governance Update*. AOP, London.

British Dental Association (2006) *Clinical Governance*. http://www.bda-dentistry.org.uk/education/education.cfm?ContentID=933.

Department of Health (1994) *Corporate Governance in the NHS, Code of Conduct, Code of Accountability*. The Stationery Office, London.

Department of Health (1997) *The New NHS: Modern, Dependable*. The Stationery Office, London.

Department of Health (1998) *A First Class Service: Quality in the new NHS*. The Stationery Office, London.

Department of Health (2000a) *The NHS Plan: A Plan for Investment, a Plan for Reform*. DH, London.

Department of Health (2003) *Building on the Best: Choice, Responsiveness and Equity in the NHS*. DH, London.

Department of Health (2004) *Standards for Better Health: Healthcare Standards for Services Under the NHS – A Consultation Document*. DH, London.

Department of Health (2006) *Integrated Governance Handbook: A Handbook for Executives and Non-executives in Healthcare Organisations*. DH, London.

Donaldson, L.J. (1998) Clinical governance: quality improvement as a duty, not a choice. *Healthcare Quality*, 4 (3) 7–9.

Emslie, S. (2001) Controls assurance in the National Health Service in England – the final piece of the corporate governance jigsaw. *Corporate Governance*, 12, March. ABG Professional Information, London.

European Region of the World Confederation for Physical Therapy (2003) *European Physiotherapy Benchmark Statement*. ERWCPT, Spain. http://www.physio-europe.org/pdf/Benchmark.pdf.

Friedman, A. (1995) Cost cuts at Barings left rogue trader unsupervised. *International Herald Tribune*, 1 March 1995. http://www.iht.com/articles/1995/03/01/risk_0.php.

Garside, P. (1999) Book review. *Clinical Governance: Making it Happen* (eds M. Lugon & J. Secker-Walker, RSM Press, London). *BMJ*, 318, 881.

Healthcare Commission (2005) *Assessment for Improvement: The Annual Health Check. Measuring What Matters.* HC, London.

Hopkins, B. (2000) National Controls Assurance Conference. *Health Care Risk Report*, 6 (3) 22–24.

Kell, J., McSherry, R. & Mudd, D. (2004) EPAS: supporting practice development. *Practice Development in Health Care*, 3 (1) 1.

McNeil, J. (1998) Clinical governance: The whys, whats, and hows for theatre practitioners. *British Journal of Theatre Nursing*, 9 (5) 208–216.

McSherry, R. (2004) Practice development and health care governance: a recipe for modernisation. *Journal of Nursing Management*, 12, 137–146.

McSherry, R. & Haddock, J. (1999) Evidence based health care: its place within clinical governance. *British Journal of Nursing*, 8 (2) 113–117.

McSherry, R. & McSherry, W. (2001) Putting research into practice. *Nursing Times*, 97, 23, 36–37.

McSherry, R. & Pearce, P.K. (2000) Interpreting the new controls guidelines. *Health Care Risk Report*, 6 (3) 19–21.

McSherry, R. & Pearce, P. (2002) *Clinical Governance: A Guide to Implementation for Healthcare Professionals.* Blackwell Science, Oxford.

McSherry, R. & Pearce, P. (2004) Healthcare standards: a critique of the Department of Health's national standards for the NHS. *Health Care Risk Report*, 10, 8 July/Aug.

NHS Executive (1999) *Health Service Circular 1999/123. Governance in the New NHS: Controls Assurance Statements 1999/2000: Risk Management and Organizational Controls.* DH, London.

NHS Executive (2001) *Health Service Circular 2001/005. Controls Assurance Statements 2000/2001 and Establishment of The Controls Assurance Support Unit.* DH, London.

Pearce, P.K. (2004) Controls assurance: benefit or burden? *Governance Matters*, 7 Aug/Sept, 5–6.

RCN (1998) *Clinical Governance: An RCN Resource Guide.* RCN, London.

Reeves, C. (2001) *Letter: Governance in the NHS.* NHS Executive, Leeds.

Royal College of General Practitioners (2005) *Royal College of General Practitioners Curriculum Statement 3.1: Clinical Governance.* RCGP, London. http://www.rcgp.org.uk/pdf/educ_clinical_governance.pdf.

Royal Pharmaceutical Society of Great Britain (2005) *What Is Clinical Governance?* RPSGB, London. http://www.rpsgb.org/members/clingov/index.html.

Scally, G. & Donaldson, L.J. (1998) Clinical governance and the drive for quality improvement in the new NHS in England. *BMJ*, 317, 4 July.

Schroeder, P.S. & Maibusch, R.M. (1984) *Nursing Quality Assurance: A Unit Based Approach.* Aspen, Rochville, Maryland.

Sealey, C. (1999) Clinical governance: an information guide for occupational therapists. *British Journal of Occupational Therapy*, 62 (6).

Smith, R. (1998) All changed, changed utterly: British medicine will be transformed by the Bristol Case. *BMJ*, 316, 1917–1918.

Stanton, P. (2004) *Making a Difference: Engaging Clinicians in PCTs.* Clinical Governance Support Team and NHS Alliance, Nottingham.

Chapter 3

A Guide to Clinical Governance

Rob McSherry and Paddy Pearce

Introduction

The previous chapters looked at the contributing factors that led to the introduction of clinical governance, and what clinical governance is. This chapter builds on the previous chapter by exploring and explaining in detail the key components of clinical governance by the application and modification of McSherry and Haddock's (1999) framework and by referring to the government's NHS Executive circulars on clinical governance and its associated components.

The key components of clinical governance

As outlined in Chapter 2, clinical governance has several themes associated with its definition: quality improvements and maintenance, professional accountability, creating and maintaining a safe environment for patients and staff, along with establishing an honest and open culture that encourages and responds to staff and public opinion – key themes for all healthcare organisations and individuals to develop in pursuit of clinical excellence.

The issue facing many healthcare organisations and individual health professionals is not in distinguishing the key themes associated with clinical governance, because we all want to practise in a clinical environment that proactively develops its staff and services in order to enhance the standards and quality of care, treatments or interventions. The concerns expressed by many healthcare professionals focus on answering the questions highlighted in Box 3.1.

Box 3.1 is not an exhaustive list of questions raised by healthcare professionals in highlighting the practicalities of developing and implementing a system of clinical governance. Box 3.1 demonstrates staff's concerns and confusions over what clinical governance has to offer at an

---

Box 3.1   Questions associated with describing the key components of clinical governance

- What are the key components of clinical governance?
- Is clinical governance only an organisational concern?
- How do you implement a system of clinical governance?
- Can a clinical governance framework be developed for individual health-care professionals to use in pursuit of clinical excellence?

---

organisational, team and individual level in improving the quality and standards of care. Essentially clinical governance is the term used to focus individual and organisational attentions back to quality 'so that quality is at the core, both of their responsibilities as organisations and of each of their staff as individual professionals' (DH 1997a, p. 47). The government's quote on clinical governance clearly responds to the questions raised in Box 3.1 by suggesting that both individual healthcare professionals and their organisations are to work within the framework of clinical governance.

Activity 3.1: Key components of clinical governance

In Chapter 2 we identified how clinical governance is about promoting, maintaining and evaluating best practices. To achieve clinical excellence at an individual and organisational level what systems or infrastructures do you feel should be in place to achieve this goal?

Write down your responses on a sheet of paper and then read on and compare your findings with those at the end of the chapter.

Before outlining the key components of clinical governance, it is essential to describe the relationship between the healthcare organisation and the achievement of quality care.

Healthcare organisations and the achievement of quality care

Clinical excellence will flourish in an organisation that proactively responds to incidents, complaints or suggestions by the public or staff regarding their experience of providing or receiving nursing care, treatments or interventions from healthcare professionals or service users. Scally and Donaldson (1998) develop the idea of quality dependence and organisational stability/instability in detail by offering an illustration that describes the variations in the quality of health by focusing on low and

Fig. 3.1   Clinical excellence and its association with organisational management styles.

high quality practices. A bell curve is offered, with low quality at one end and high quality at the other. Where low or poor quality is experienced, potential problems could exist in the form of untoward incidents and increased complaints; the aim is for healthcare organisations to shift changes in practice from the centre or mean towards the high quality. Whilst the Scally and Donaldson (1998) illustration outlining the variations in the quality of health organisations is a useful way of viewing the standards of quality, it is not without its limitations. For example, how does an organisation establish the mean or best practices for a certain service? How does the organisation or individual know that the standards of practice are of high or low quality?

To address some of the above limitations and to further build on Scally and Donaldson's (1998) work it is important to demonstrate the link between proactive and reactionary organisational management in achieving clinical excellence, and its association with implementing a clinical governance framework, as depicted in Fig. 3.1.

It is clear from Fig. 3.1 that a system of clinical governance will only be achieved where a balance between reactionary and proactive management exists within the healthcare organisation; this will hopefully result in the continued provision of medium to high quality care. To achieve high quality care it is essential that the right culture and clinical environments and services are created, and this depends on nurturing a proactive approach to management. That is not to say reactionary management is ineffective, because there may be occasions when this type of approach is advocated. To create an open culture that positively seeks and responds to criticisms and compliments will take time, but it is the preferred style advocated within the clinical governance frameworks.

So what are the qualities required by an organisation to become more proactive in nature? Scally and Donaldson (1998) and Donaldson and Muir Gray (1998) indicate that quality improvements are dependent on having an:

'organisation-wide approach to quality improvement with emphasis on preventing adverse outcomes through simplification and improving the process of care. Leadership and commitment from the top of the organisation, team work, consumer focus, and good data are also important.' (Scally & Donaldson 1998, p. 62)

These are key attributes inferred by having a proactive management approach.

The White Paper *The New NHS: Modern, Dependable* (DH 1997a) described how a quality organisation can be achieved by proactively ensuring that the ten attributes and processes shown in Box 3.2 are present.

Box 3.2 Key attributes associated with promotion of a quality organisation

- There is an integrated approach to quality improvement throughout the whole organisation.
- Leadership skills are developed in line with professional and clinical needs.
- Infrastructures exist that foster the development of evidence-based practices.
- Innovations are valued and good practices are shared within and without the organisation.
- Clinical risk management systems are in place.
- There is a proactive approach to reporting and dealing with and learning from untoward incidents.
- Complaints are taken seriously and actions taken to prevent any recurrence.
- Poor clinical performance is recognised, thus preventing potential harm to patients or staff.
- Practice and professional development is aligned and integral to clinical governance frameworks.
- Clinical data are of the best quality and can be used effectively to monitor patient care and clinical outcomes.

Adapted from DH (1997a)

It is evident from Box 3.2 that the establishment of a proactive organisational culture is dependent on the development of 'effective channels of communication between healthcare professionals' (McSherry

& Haddock 1999) and infrastructures such as education, training, research and access to high quality information in supporting staff in their pursuit of clinical excellence. Essentially, 'successful quality improvement demands major cultural change – but that change cannot simply be imposed, as it entails a significant shift in the way that people think and behave' (Walshe *et al.* 2000, p. 1). The question that often remains unanswered in much of the literature reviewed by the authors is, how do you achieve successful culture change(s)?

Figure 3.1 demonstrates how a proactive management style is the best way to promote an honest and open culture, which can and will only be achieved through strong leadership and commitment to genuine quality improvement. This approach to management, of openly encouraging a shared ownership for the active development, implementation and evaluation of the infrastructures associated with clinical governance, is the key to success. Involvement of staff from all levels within and without the organisation needs to be carefully considered. Without the involvement and cooperation of clinical staff, clinical governance will not make a difference to patient care.

A possible approach for encouraging positive cultural shifts or changes in attitudes is that offered by McSherry and Haddock (1999) in highlighting the key components and structures of evidence-based practice (see Fig. 3.2).

Figure 3.2 describes how the development of staff culture is paramount if successful implementation of evidence-based practice in relation to clinical governance is to be achieved. The key components are the

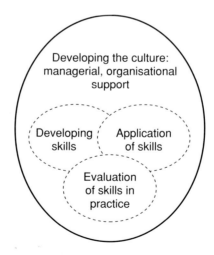

Fig. 3.2 Promoting a culture for evidence-based practice within clinical governance. (Reproduced from McSherry and Haddock (1999) with kind permission of Mark Allen Publishing Ltd.)

development, application and evaluation of practices that can be used at organisational and individual levels.

The same approach could be transferred to the development of clinical governance in that the correct organisational culture needs to be established whilst the infrastructures are being developed and implemented. The starting point for healthcare organisations to successfully implement clinical governance is to review the White Papers (DH 1997a, 1998), Department of Health guidance documents and NHS Circular 1999/065 (NHS Executive 1999a) on clinical governance with reference to local internal organisational structures and policies.

It is evident from the information presented thus far that clinical governance is a highly complex system containing and involving many themes and management and organisational processes in the pursuit of individual and organisational clinical quality. What remains to be described and discussed is how to ensure that clinical governance becomes a reality for all practising healthcare professionals, NHS personnel and healthcare organisations.

Upon reading the NHS Circular 1999/065 and the literature by Edwards and Packham (1999), McSherry and Haddock (1999) and Donaldson (2000), several key themes emerge that encompass the key elements of clinical governance (Fig. 3.3). It is evident from Fig. 3.3

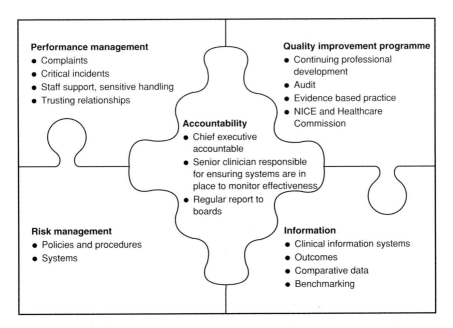

Fig. 3.3 Key components of clinical governance. (Modified from the McSherry & Haddock (1999) template outlining clinical governance.)

that risk management, performance management, quality improvement, information and accountability are central to the delivery of clinical governance. This will now be outlined in more detail.

Risk management

Risk management simply means practising safely: 'It aims to develop good practice and reduce the occurrence of harmful or adverse incidents' (RCN 2000, p. 19). The concept of risk management is about the reduction of clinical and non-clinical risks associated with healthcare. In the past, risk management focused on the financial areas of healthcare. It is important to remember when exploring the notion of risk that the following definitions of risk could be applied to either the clinical or non-clinical aspects of healthcare:

- A variation in the outcomes that could occur over a specified period in a given situation (Williams & Heins 1976).
- The possibility of incurring misfortune or loss (Collins 1985).
- The chance or possibility of bad outcome (Wilson & Tingle 1999).
- The probability or likelihood that harm may occur, coupled with the consequences of that harm (Mayatt 2004).

Healthcare governance is about the management of 'risk' regardless of its origins within the corporate systems and processes. Some healthcare professionals, teams and organisations tend to view 'risk' in relation to their own position and profession and not in a holistic manner; this may result in only partial reductions and minimisations of a given risk, which may be seen only as a clinical risk. Clinical risk is defined as 'a clinical error to be at variance from intended treatment, care, therapeutic intervention or diagnostic result; there may be an untoward outcome or not' (Wilson & Tingle 1999, p. 71). This notion is evidenced in the following example. Several patients in a specific clinical area develop wound infections resulting in extended lengths of stay, patient discomfort and increased workload and costs for staff working in that organisation. If this situation was identified by a clinician as a professional issue only, he or she might identify the clinical risk but fail to consider the broader issues surrounding this situation, such as ward cleanliness, adherence to infection control policies and procedures, addressing education and training, and overall considerations of resource allocation and finance.

Risk management is mainly 'concerned with harnessing the information and expertise of individuals within the organisation and translating that with their help into positive action which will reduce loss of life, financial loss, loss of staff availability, loss of the availability of buildings or equipment and loss of reputation' (DH 1994). Within the context of healthcare governance the identification and management of risks should be viewed in a holistic way associated with the clinical, environmental and operational aspects of the incident, situation or event.

However, the most important aspect, that of clinical quality, has been underdeveloped (DH 2000a). This philosophy over the past few years has changed significantly. It would seem that since the lifting of crown immunity in 1995, where central government was responsible for the payment of clinical negligence claims for all NHS organisations, a shift in responsibility to the individual NHS organisations has occurred for the settlement of such claims. This change in policy has made NHS organisations seriously consider how their organisation and staff are managing risks. In response to the lifting of crown immunity, NHS Trusts realised the need to address this issue of protecting themselves from the pursuit of clinical negligence claims which would have to be financed from their annual budgets.

The lifting of crown immunity led to the establishment of the Clinical Negligence Scheme for Trusts (CNST) in 1995. The basic principle of the scheme is similar to a personal, household or car insurance where you pay your premiums and obtain discounts for no-claims. With CNST you pay your premiums based on the size of your hospital, its specialties, and on your claims history, and you receive discount for minimising and managing clinical risks. The level of discount is associated with achieving compliance with standards ranging from level one to three. The higher the level of accreditation against the required standards, the greater the discount. Essentially the CNST is a pooling scheme for its members where, should a huge negligence claim be made against a Trust, the scheme would pay out the settlement after the Trust had paid its excess (Mayatt 1995). The standards are concerned with having (NHSLA 2005):

- A clinical risk strategy.
- An identified executive director responsible for the management of clinical risk.
- A system for reporting, monitoring and evaluating clinical incidents and near misses (i.e. a potentially harmful incident that could have had adverse consequences for a patient/carer).
- A major clinical incident policy, e.g. to address an infectious disease outbreak or medical equipment failure.
- A system for complaints reporting, monitoring and actioning.
- Available consent and advice policies, i.e. patients are informed of the risks and benefits of a procedure from an individual capable of doing that procedure.

- Policies for the recording, storing and auditing of all patient records.
- Systems for induction training and the ongoing development of professional competence.
- Clinical standards for the promotion of clinical quality pertinent to specialty groups, e.g. maternity, mental health and ambulance, and new combined schemes to cover Primary Care Trusts.

The CNST offers a framework to minimise and manage clinical risks in the pursuit of clinical excellence. Initially CNST was intended to reduce financial risks: 'a large settlement or a series of sizable settlements could significantly impinge upon the overall financial position of a Trust' (Mayatt 1995, p. 2). Today CNST is a voluntary scheme administered by the NHS Litigation Authority that supports the clinical risk aspect of clinical governance. However, there continues to be room for ongoing development and improving the clinical risk infrastructures, as alluded to by the Chief Medical Officer (DH 2000a). An example of improved clinical risk infrastructures could be the establishment of a national incident reporting system to detect potential clinical risks for all NHS organisations at an early stage.

This approach to the management of risks was highlighted in *An Organisation with a Memory* (DH 2000a) and how it will be actioned via *Building a Safer NHS for Patents: Implementing an Organisation with a Memory* (DH 2001). Following the publication of these documents, the National Patient Safety Agency (NPSA) was established in July 2001 with a remit of improving patient safety by enabling organisations and individuals to learn from the experiences of others. The NPSA has tackled the limitations highlighted by *Organisation with a Memory* (DH 2000a) by publishing several safety bulletins concerned with protecting patients from harm. These include *Patient Alert 02* (NPSA 2004), where all NHS hospitals in England use a universal telephone number (2222). Similarly, the NPSA has removed injectable forms of potassium that used to be added to intravenous solutions for transfusion (NPSA 2003a). The NPSA has introduced the National Reporting and Learning System (NRLS) (NPSA 2003b) which gathers and disseminates learning from patient safety incidents. The NPSA also provides relevant advice and guidance regarding Root Cause Analysis (RCA). RCA is designed to capture, review and disseminate lessons learnt from patient safety incidents. Despite the progress made by the NPSA, the National Audit Office (NAO) argues that more still needs to be done by this agency (NAO 2005). The NAO is a national body with the remit of scrutinising public services on behalf of the United Kingdom (UK) parliament. The purpose is to ensure that public money is spent prudently.

It is important to mention here that whilst the CNST standards have done much to advance risk management and reduce clinical risks, a need for a holistic management of 'risk' has been introduced via the controls assurance standards (www.doh.gov/riskman.htm), which further enhance a whole systems approach towards risk management within the NHS in England. These are standards to which all healthcare organisations must adhere. The National Health Service Litigation Authority (NHSLA) which runs the CNST scheme also runs the non-clinical schemes for the NHS, namely liability to third parties and property essences (NHSLA 2006). Put simply these could be paralleled to insuring your personal property and belongings. The NHSLA combines the two schemes into one framework for Primary Care Trusts (PCT) and has produced the risk management standard for PCTs. Similarly to the CNST, the greater the compliance with the standards, the greater the reduction in premiums paid. To ensure compliance with these standards NHS organisations need to adopt a strategic and systematic approach to managing performance.

Managing performance

The DH (1997a) reforms of the NHS provided a performance assessment framework that supports the drive for higher quality standards by ensuring that performance assessment is focused on the delivery of effective, appropriate and timely healthcare services which meet local needs (DH 1997a, p. 63).

Within the clinical governance framework the management of poor performance of either devices or personnel is imperative in reducing clinical failures. As highlighted earlier in this chapter, management styles play an important part in how people perform. In addition to having a proactive management style and an honest and open culture which encourages staff and the public to express ideas or concerns, how can an organisation detect, promote and deal with good or poor performance?

It is acknowledged within the literature (DH 2000a; RCN 2000) that the delivery of healthcare involves many complex processes involving many individuals to provide the best service to the public. With this in mind it is easier to apportion blame to individuals rather than the systems when things go wrong. This is because for many organisations, reviewing systems is time consuming and costly, and for some organisations it is about establishing where to start. The easy option is to blame the individual when things go wrong, but this reactionary approach is not beneficial to preventing recurrence of the situation. What is needed is a review of the systems and processes associated with the incident, and to be honest and open with the findings. This proactive approach to dealing with incidents or complaints involving individuals, teams or processes requires a major cultural shift, as eloquently described by the Royal College of Nursing:

> 'A culture that encourages open discussion and reflection on practice allows staff to learn from their experiences. This includes both celebrating what is done well and learning from what is done less well. However, if an organisation is going to encourage clinicians to report incidents and learn from mistakes, it must develop a blame free culture, rather than one that revolves around disciplinary procedures.' (RCN 2000, p. 8)

It is evident from the RCN's definition that performance management in healthcare services needs to be reorganised to deal with good and poor performances, as this has not been the case in the past. Achieving this goal is about developing simple but effective systems and processes that capture the performances of individuals, teams, organisations and devices that work well and not so well. The overall aim of this type of performance management is to establish, share and learn from the experiences of others.

Activity 3.2: Performance management

Write down what you think influences the performance of an individual, team or organisation along with the systems and processes that should be developed in an organisation to assist in dealing with good or poor performance.

Compare your responses with those in the feedback box at the end of the chapter.

We believe that two main factors influence performance management in the NHS: the perceived experiences of the public and the organisation's philosophical approach to performance. Figure 3.4 provides a framework outlining the various components associated with performance management, of which more is explained below.

Figure 3.4 shows how performance management is about dealing with good and not so good performance. It is clear that the public's view is based upon individuals' experiences of, or the media coverage of, the services or a combination of both. Often 'all that is good in healthcare is regarded by the public as being attributable to doctors and nurses, while all that is bad is the fault of managers and their political masters' (Baker 1998, p. 137). The quote by Baker is plausible and in most cases true, but for performance management to operate effectively within the context of clinical governance frameworks, this perception needs to be challenged.

Fig. 3.4   Framework for performance management.

Baker's quote seems to suggest that the public and perhaps many health service staff fail to understand that performance depends on uniting the non-clinical infrastructures with the clinical, along with the processes and systems associated with each. Poor performance can often be the result of systems and process failure rather than individuals or vice versa.

Systems are only as good as the design: if this is ineffective then so is the information or care given as a result. To develop good performance management systems within the context of clinical governance in Acute and Mental Health Trusts, Primary Care Trusts, Ambulance Trusts, Foundation Trusts and Strategic Health Authorities, boards need to embrace a philosophy that proactively encourages the concept of performance management. In a simple way they need to be able to answer three questions: What are we doing? How well are we doing it? And how do we know we are performing well? These can only be answered by having the appropriate systems in place to collect and disseminate information associated with good and not so good performance related to the clinical and non-clinical aspects of healthcare service.

Figure 3.4 shows that there are several systems and processes that need to be in place to provide information on performance. Performance needs to be considered in line with a whole systems approach, where clinical performance and non-clinical performance are seen as equal (McSherry 2004). In the past the NHS has tended to focus on financial performance and activity, i.e. the number of patient treatments and length of waiting lists. This information is important and needs to be collected; however, it does not provide managers or the public with any information about the quality of care and services provided or indeed how individuals or systems are performing. An example of this is an individual who could be seen within the maximum four-hour waiting time in an Accident and Emergency Department. However, there may be limited information gathered regarding the patient experience, quality of the service provided and eventual clinical outcome of the patient.

A range of quality indicators need to be developed that provide information and evidence on either individual, team or organisational performance. These systems and associated processes need to capture activity from a variety of sources, i.e. organisational, team and individual performance such as pressure sore prevalence, hospital-acquired infections, patient satisfaction, and clinical outcomes. If we apply these examples to Fig. 3.4 it is evident how systems such as clinical incident reporting, complaints and accolades monitoring, financial and quality reporting, performance reviews and the recording of sickness and absence can demonstrate the overall performance of individuals, teams and the organisation. This is because each part of the performance management system includes reviewing and acting on the information given in demonstrating good or not so good practice, which can be highlighted through pooling information gathered from several systems and processes such as described below.

Clinical incident reporting

Clinical incident reporting is required for staff and patients in highlighting any areas where an individual or organisation fails to deliver the appropriate standard of care. Incident reporting offers a framework for the detection of untoward incidents and near misses, which enables action to be taken, lessons to be learnt, practices to be reviewed and information to be shared to prevent any recurrence.

Individual performance review

Individual performance review (IPR) should encourage staff to express and report any concerns about their own individual practices so that continued improvements can be made in the delivery of services and in promoting safe practice. Following an IPR a personal development plan (PDP) should be written and agreed by the parties to enable the individual and department to develop their practices in line with the overall direction of the employing organisation (Martin 2000). With the introduction of the Agenda for Change (AfC) (DH 2004a) and the Knowledge and Skills Framework (KSF) (DH 2004b), pay is linked to performance. For a member of staff to progress to the next increment of the scale he or she needs to demonstrate achievement of the competencies agreed in the KSF for the post he/she holds. This again reaffirms the importance of having an IPR and a PDP.

Complaints and accolades monitoring

Complaints and accolades monitoring elicits trends and patterns in care delivery, enabling the most appropriate action to be taken or indeed to celebrate areas of good performance.

Sickness and absence monitoring

Sickness and absence monitoring enables either the individual, teams or organisation to evaluate the well-being of personnel and can be used to help explain areas of poor performance, e.g. rising numbers of clinical complaints in a ward area because of staff shortages due to sickness and absence. The DH is beginning to realise the importance of investing in staff and in creating a sound working environment and good working relationships. The work of West *et al.* (2000) showed a relationship between staff morale, job satisfaction and mortality. Perhaps this work influenced the development of the Improving Working Lives (IWL) initiative introduced by the DH (DH 2000b). Taking West *et al.* (2000) and the DH (2000b) work into account it would seem that organisations with higher levels of staff satisfaction and morale have better patient outcomes than NHS organisations with lower levels of staff satisfaction and morale.

   In summary, performance management is about the integration and utilisation of data and information obtained from services often viewed with negative connotations, such as clinical incident reporting, complaints and clinical audit. However, these systems and processes should be viewed positively, because they often demonstrate the existence of quality services and standards of practice. Performance management is about the integration of the various systems and sources of information in highlighting the overall quality status of the organisation (Garland 1998).

Quality improvement

'Clinical governance' is about assuring sustainable continuous quality improvement, which can only be achieved by the determined and conscious

Fig. 3.5   Continuous quality improvement: the route to clinical excellence.

efforts of the clinical and non-clinical staff who have the appropriate support of their organisation to deliver best practice. To obtain improvements in quality systems there needs to be in place appropriate support to
facilitate individuals and organisations in the pursuit of clinical excellence
(NHS Executive 1999a). Continuous quality improvement is the route to
clinical excellence. Clinical excellence can only be achieved by having
efficient and effective systems of communication with staff and patients
and where infrastructures are established that proactively seek to develop,
maintain and monitor the standards and quality of care provided by
the organisation and individuals themselves. The words 'vigilant' and
'surveillance' come to mind in ensuring that the term clinical governance
becomes an integral part of all daily practices.

Figure 3.5 highlights how clinical excellence can be achieved by having an
organisation that continually seeks to improve its standards and practices
by having integrated systems of clinical risk management, clinical audit,
and practices based on sound evidence-based research, which form the
basis of staff development. It becomes apparent from Fig. 3.5 that quality
improvement is based around the following robust systems and processes:

- Clinical risk management and clinical audit.
- Continued practice and professional development.

- Implementing continuing professional development within an NHS organisation.
- Research and development.
- Evidence-based healthcare.

Clinical risk management and clinical audit

As outlined previously in this chapter, risk management is about the development of robust systems which assist staff in establishing efficient and effective standards of care against local, national or international standards, in an attempt to minimise and proactively manage risks.

Clinical audit is defined as the systematic and critical review of systems and processes of care, a method that is essential in order to compare performance against evidence-based standards, for example compliance with National Institute for Health and Clinical Excellence (NICE) guidelines. NICE has been responsible for the appraisal and assessment of new and existing technologies and for producing guidelines for the NHS. Clinical audit is the tool to measure compliance of treatment, interventions or care offered to patients, and the resulting effectiveness on patient care. Areas of poor practice or potential risk should be highlighted so that standards or local policies and guidelines can be written to prevent incidents or harm to patients.

Continued practice and professional development

To ensure that an organisation and staff deliver a high quality service, they need to have sound knowledge and well developed skills and competencies to perform their roles efficiently and effectively. Lifelong learning and continuing professional development (CPD) should be seen as an ongoing process in ensuring that practices are the most effective and up to date. The term CPD was originally mentioned in the government's White Papers (DH 1997a, 1998), where the government set out its long-term goal of modernising the NHS, with the key focus for change centred on quality improvements. In order to achieve this, healthcare organisations must have robust systems and processes to ensure the continued professional development of all their employees.

CPD is defined as:

'A process of lifelong learning for all individuals and teams which meets the needs of patients and delivers the health outcomes and healthcare priorities of the NHS and which enables professionals to expand and fulfil their potential.' (DH 1998, p. 42)

CPD should be seen as the beginning of a process of developing a culture of lifelong learning for all staff. To develop a robust system and process for the delivery of CPD, local ownership is essential. We do recognise that this is a long-term objective, will take several years to achieve and requires the backing from the chairs and chief executives of healthcare organisations because they have a key role to play in ensuring CPD via collaboration and communication between managers, human resources, nursing and medical education committees, and in ensuring that the educational aspect of CPD meets their organisation's and professional staff's requirements. CPD is for all parts of the NHS; with the increasingly competitive labour market the NHS needs to pay attention to the development of managers and information technology personnel in order to ensure access to current information in supporting the development of their employees and services. To facilitate the development of a system for CPD within a healthcare organisation or team or for individuals, it is imperative to action the points outlined in the Health Service Circular 1999/154 Continuing Professional Development: Quality in the New NHS (NHS Executive 1999b). To illustrate how this can be achieved, the following example is taken from Pearce and McSherry (2000).

Implementing continuing professional development within an NHS organisation

In order to implement HSC 1999/154 within the NHS, individual organisations need to adopt a focused approach to ensure the delivery of high quality care, an approach that could be enhanced by the development of robust CPD. In applying this principle the concept of 'management' by objectives could be introduced. This style of managing CPD enables Trusts to anticipate and highlight important issues relevant to the needs of their healthcare population. Corporate objectives are set prior to the start of the financial year, which are specific to the core elements of the organisation's business plan. From these core objectives, sub-objectives for clinical and general managers are established and linked to the personal development plans (PDP) for their staff. A PDP is linked to the individual's annual performance appraisal where the employee and manager review the year's progress and assess strengths, weaknesses, opportunities and threats (SWOT analysis), jointly agreeing a personal development plan for the next twelve months with a six-monthly review. This approach enables the Trust to systematically identify the important national, regional and local issues to inform a coherent and coordinated strategy in achieving the objectives. This approach to CPD ensures that the Trust is working collaboratively as a team. Figure 3.6 illustrates a model of the CPD processes.

Phase 1	February/March
Corporate objectives to executive directors	

Phase 2	April
Executive and general clinical managers agree objectives to address corporate objectives	

Phase 3	April
General and clinical managers and heads of department agree objectives of their respective departments	

Phase 4	April
Employees and line managers agree individual objectives and personal development plans in line with the Knowledge and Skills Framework (DH 2004b)	

Fig. 3.6   A model to aid the facilitation of CPD into healthcare organisations.

CPD will be discussed in more detail in Chapter 4. This is related to case study 3 and personal and professional development plans. It is also worth noting here that CPD is a key element of the Investors in People Award, to which many healthcare organisations and teams aspire (for more information on this award visit the website http://www.iip.co.uk). CPD also forms a major part of the NHS Improving Working Lives (IWL) standard (DH 2000b), which all NHS organisations need to attain. It is evident from the above information that CPD and lifelong learning are integral aspects of the clinical governance framework and can only be achieved by mutual collaboration, respect, openness and honesty between employees and employers over how the individual and the organisation are performing. Successful implementation of clinical governance depends on adequate resourcing and genuine commitment from all parties involved, i.e. from the DH to the individual member of staff.

Research and development (R&D)

Research and development is an integral part of clinical governance. The 'R' (research) aspect is often associated with the generation of new, and testing of existing, knowledge. The 'D' (development) aspect is often unsupported and undervalued in many healthcare organisations, e.g. within clinical governance, staff are expected to be research aware, although little resource is allocated to support this need (McSherry *et al.* 2006). One aspect of R&D is concerned with establishing ways of enhancing health by the introduction of research. For more information on R&D view the DH Research and Development website: http://www.dh.gov.uk/research. To promote evidence-based practice a system for accessing, implementing, monitoring, supporting, supervising and disseminating research findings should be established to ensure that clinical practices and patient care are based on the most recent and best available scientific evidence, commonly referred to as evidence-based practice. So what is evidence-based practice? The following sections are based on McSherry and Haddock (1999) with kind permission of Mark Allen Publishers Ltd.

Evidence-based healthcare

Evidence-based practice is 'the process of systematically finding and using contemporaneous research findings as the basis for clinical decision-making' (Long & Harrison 1996) and is an integral part of the clinical governance framework, as illustrated in Figs 3.2 and 3.5. For the successful implementation of clinical governance for organisations and individuals, it is essential that all systems, processes, infrastructures and health professionals are developed using the principles of evidence-based practice. To facilitate the development of evidence-based practice the following processes need to be applied (Kitson 1997; Cullum *et al.* 1998; Swage 1998; McSherry *et al.* 2001):

- Identify areas in practice from which clear clinical questions can be formulated.
- Identify the best-related evidence from available literature.
- Critically appraise the evidence for validity and clinical usefulness.
- Implement and incorporate relevant findings into practice.
- Subsequently measure performance against expected outcomes or against peers.
- Ensure staff are supported and developed through adequate resourcing of evidence-based practice, education and training programmes.

For example, to develop an evidence-based organisational strategy for clinical risk management, in ensuring the systematic delivery of appropriate and safe healthcare by the organisation and all its employees, healthcare professionals require regular clinical exposure and experience (Cullum *et al.* 1998). This is essential in order for them to become familiar and competent in rationalising the risks and benefits of a particular treatment, intervention or delivery of care, to deal with the patient's unique individual set of circumstances. It should only be allowed to occur following a structured period of education and supervision, and when the individual feels competent to do the procedure without assistance.

The continued clinical exposure, observations and experience of new treatments or interventions should in addition be supported by the relevant research evidence, where patient participation is reflected in the final choice of treatment, intervention or application of care. The development of healthcare professionals able to equip themselves with the critical appraisal skills required to rationalise the risks and benefits of care, and indeed to critique research evidence, requires organisational leadership and service support, sufficient resources and indeed a change in the culture to enable staff to work in this way. Therefore in order for evidence-based practice to function within the context of clinical governance and to truly exist and operate effectively, the key components and structures illustrated in Fig. 3.2 are required.

Figure 3.2 illustrates that it is essential that efficient and effective channels of communication and information-giving are established in order to promote a culture that proactively develops infrastructures that nurture professional and practice development in the pursuit of clinical excellence (Rycroft-Malone *et al.* 2004). This can only be achieved by ensuring that the services provided are staffed by appropriately skilled, knowledgeable and competent practitioners, who are then actively supported in order to further develop, apply and evaluate the care or service provided, with the aim of improving the quality and standards of care and treatment delivered to patients. McCormack *et al.* (2004) argue that evidence-based practice is dependent on the creation of an appropriate environment and culture, which facilitates the development of evidence-based care. This approach makes it essential for healthcare professionals to know how and where to access and appraise the evidence.

Locating the evidence

The following is a guide to where research evidence may be obtained in supporting clinical practices:

- Libraries (local and national)
- Voluntary and support organisations
- Clinical audit departments
- Centres for research and development
- Practice development centres
- Centre for Reviews and Dissemination (York)
- Professional bodies
- Local universities
- Information technology centres

- Electronic computerised databases (CINHAL, MEDLINE)
- The Cochrane Library
- The National Electronic Library for Health (NeLH)
- Expert advice

A fundamental problem facing some healthcare professionals after obtaining the relevant information or research evidence is the process of critical appraisal, i.e. how do you evaluate the information? Is it useful, reliable and relevant? This was highlighted by Swage (1998), who states that 'many nurses (indeed all health professionals) stumble at the first hurdle because they are not confident about understanding research and reviews'.

Evidence-based care and the need for critical appraisal skills

Crombie (1996), Sackett *et al.* (1997) and Swage (1998) suggest that critical appraisal is about considering the relevance of a research question, evaluating the evidence collected to answer the question, and assessing the effectiveness of the conclusion and the recommendation of the evidence. In a simple way it is about systematically reviewing and questioning the stages of the research process, i.e. title and abstract, introduction/literature review, methods, results, discussions and recommendations, and asking the following questions (adapted from Crombie 1996):

- Is the research of interest?
- Why was it done?
- How was it performed?
- Who was it done to?
- What did it show?
- What is the possible implication for your practice?
- What next: information only, uninteresting or support practice?

Having had the education and training to critically appraise research, in the hope of practising evidence-based care, why is it that so many healthcare professionals continue to base practice around tradition or rituals despite research evidence showing the contrary? Perhaps this is because of some of the barriers to implementation.

Barriers to implementation of the evidence

An enormous amount of literature continues to flood the academic journals relating to all professional groups, suggesting that the theory–practice gap continues to widen (May *et al.* 1998; Pallen & Timmins 2002; Glacken 2004). To instigate evidence-based care at a clinical level, perhaps organisations and staff need to become familiar with these barriers and begin to develop realistic strategies to overcome them. Healthcare professionals need to challenge these barriers in the continued attempt to improve their quality and standards of clinical practices in the light of rising patient expectations and recent government reforms (see Chapter 1).

The barriers that continue to be faced by many are as follows:

- Attitudes towards research
- Lack of confidence, understanding and the skills to critically appraise
- Insufficient time within work commitments
- Lack of support from peers, managers and other health professionals
- Lack of resources
- Resistance to change

Despite attempts to implement research evidence to support practices, many staff continue to experience difficulty with ensuring that the care and treatment they provide is evaluated effectively. Barriers are explored in more detail in Chapter 5.

Evaluation of the evidence

It is important that, following the implementation of research findings on delivering care and treatments, we continue to evaluate the quality, standard and effectiveness of our intervention with regards to patient outcomes or benefits to the service or organisation. There are many ways in addition to peer review that this can be achieved:

- Clinical audit
- Comparing standards against national guidance, e.g. NICE, Scottish Intercollegiate Guidelines Network (SIGN), Royal Colleges Guidelines
- Using a performance management framework
- Benchmarking: the use of comparative performance, i.e. comparing standards and outcomes against similar organisations
- Involvement in National Audits performed by the Royal College of Physicians on stroke and continence care
- Improvement reviews and performance against Standards for Better Health undertaken by the Healthcare Commission

In summary, should efficient and effective systems of continuous professional development, research and development, clinical risk and clinical audit be established, the overall cultural emphasis shifts from a reactive nature – i.e. acting on complaints from an unfortunate incident or an area of poor practice or performance resulting from either an individual or service failure – to a more proactive nature, in trying to avoid the incident from happening in the first place (McSherry & Haddock 1999).

Quality information

In order to make continuous quality improvement in organisations, teams and individuals, quality information is needed. For healthcare professionals and organisations to deliver quality standards, effective communication and information-giving are essential. Communication is defined as 'the exchange of information for some purposes' (McCabe & Timmins 2006). This broad definition of communication is pertinent when exploring clinical governance because it emphasises the enormous task in hand for all healthcare professionals in tailoring their services to the client group and clinical setting and in exchanging the relevant information with patients, carers, the public and fellow professionals. Information-giving refers to 'the knowledge acquired through experience or study' (Collins 1985). To provide quality information healthcare professionals need to have the knowledge, understanding and effective communication skills to exchange and receive information with and from their patients, carers and colleagues. The Audit Commission (1992) acknowledged that healthcare organisations and processes are complex, reinforcing the need for effective communication with patients about the clinical and non-clinical aspects of care. The report stated that 'lack of information and problems in communicating with health professionals usually come at the top of patients' concerns' (Audit Commission 1992), an issue that continues to remain current. To address the concerns of patients and indeed the public with regard to poor communication and information-giving, many government initiatives have been introduced to improve communications within the NHS (Box 3.3). Furthermore, the Picker Institute Europe has a wealth of information about patient experience. See their website for more details (www.pickereurope.org).

Box 3.3 Government initiatives aimed at improving communication and information giving

- *The Patient's Charter: Raising the Standards* (DH 1992a)
- *The Citizen's Charter* (DH 1992b)
- *Code of Openness in the NHS* (DH 1997b)
- Data Protection Act 1998
- Health Service Circular 1999/053, *For the Record: Managing Records in NHS Trusts and Health Authorities* (NHS Executive 1999c)
- *Information for Health* (NHS Executive 2000a)
- The Caldicott Report (NHS Executive 2000b)
- *Our Health, Our Care, Our Say* (DH 2006a)

When referring to Box 3.3 and reflecting upon these documents it is easy to see the importance the government is placing on communication and information-giving in an effort to address the issues surrounding poor communication and the stress and anxiety this causes patients and professionals alike. Effective communications are an integral aspect of clinical governance; furthermore, communication within and between the key processes is vital in ensuring quality services. Communication and information-giving can be enhanced by auditing communications processes along with paying attention to the quality of information provided. In the *Code of Openness in the NHS* (DH 1997b) the principles of good communication and information-giving are provided based around access to information, explanations, reasons for decisions and actions, and information about what data are available. We believe that information should be given as outlined in Box 3.4.

Box 3.4   Principles of effective information giving

The information must be:

- Accurate: factually correct.
- Timely: given at the right stage of the process or intervention required.
- Current: up to date with appropriate evidence.
- Easily accessible: provided in several formats, i.e. computer based, leaflets.
- Clear and concise: simple and easy to understand or follow.
- Audience specific: to consider ethnicity, disability, and be provided in a sensitive manner.
- Relevant: focused and specific detail.

Note: when producing patient information leaflets or when sending information to patients, the Plain English Society could be contacted or any other relevant organisations such as the Charter Mark.

It is evident from Boxes 3.3 and 3.4 and the previous paragraphs that communication and information are important aspects in ensuring clinical excellence for patients, as well as being essential factors for the successful implementation, monitoring and evaluation of clinical governance systems and processes. To demonstrate the effectiveness of clinical governance arrangements within healthcare organisations, information and communication are vital.

Information requirements for effective clinical governance systems

Quality information within the clinical governance framework is essential and information needs to be considered at four levels within the NHS:

healthcare organisations, teams and individuals (healthcare professionals and patients).

Healthcare organisations

As clinical governance is about sustained improvement in the care provided by the health service there is a requirement to demonstrate that this is happening. To do this, a vast amount of clinical and non-clinical information is required. The Commission for Health Improvement (CHI) had the responsibility for reviewing the clinical governance arrangements of NHS Trusts, Health Authorities and Primary Care Trusts (PCTs). CHI originally planned to perform clinical governance reviews (CGR) on a four year cycle, i.e. to review clinical governance in all NHS organisations every four years. An important aspect of CHI's CGR is the analysis of information provided by the organisation. CHI was disbanded in 2003 and its role of critically reviewing the performance of NHS organisation transferred to the Commission for Healthcare Audit and Inspection, commonly known today as the Healthcare Commission (HC). During its lifespan CHI carried out CGRs in the majority of NHS organisations in England, along with undertaking a number of investigations (CHI 2004). These can be broadly summarised into service failures and inappropriate professional behaviours (CHI 2004). Since the introduction of the HC, two principal aims have emerged: to reduce the burden of inspection upon the NHS and to make review and inspection more targeted and proportionate. The HC intends to do this by the use of intelligent information, i.e. using performance information that currently exists gathered by reviews and inspections performed by other agencies and regulators such as the NHSLA, Audit Commission (AC) and the Health and Safety Executive (HSE) to name but a few.

To meet the challenges posed by the introduction of clinical governance we suggest that clinical governance leads in Trusts read and reflect upon these HC documents and use them as a basis for the development of the Trust's information strategies and in supporting their clinical governance frameworks. Further information is available at www.healthcarecommission.org.uk.

Clinical teams

To facilitate clinical governance at the clinical team level, all clinical teams need information on how well they are performing. The type of data and information required to support this process can be categorised into those associated with quantitative (numerical/statistical information) and qualitative (patient and staffing experience) or a combination of both; for example, with complaints reporting you need numbers and trends to detect patterns, and also qualitative information about individual complaints or letters of commendation. Likewise this could apply to infection control issues. Examples of quantitative and qualitative information are as follows:

- *Activity*: numbers of patients treated, e.g. finished consultant episodes (FCEs), average length of stay (LOS).
- *Quality*: quality indicators (QI), incidence of infections, complaints, pressure sore prevalence rates.
- *Outcome measures*: data pertaining to improved quality of life for the patient with regard to, e.g. mobility, pain, which is obtained from the use of validated measurement tools, e.g. SF36, Hospital Anxiety Depression Scale, Barthel Index.
- *Readmissions*: these could be unplanned, i.e. patients returning to ITU, CCU, or discharged patients being readmitted soon after discharge.
- *Clinical incidents*: any untoward incident that can potentially affect the patient's outcome, e.g. drug errors, breakdowns in communication affecting patient care, inappropriate care.
- Health and safety incidents: e.g. falls, accidents at work, moving and handling for staff and patients.
- *Benchmarking*: comparative information between similar clinical and non-clinical teams regarding team performance in standards and quality of care, e.g. stroke audit, UK Trauma and Audit Network, Standards for Better Health (DH 2004c).
- *Accreditation*: verification of the standards and quality of care/ interventions against set standards, e.g. the King's Fund accreditation website www.kingsfund.org.uk or the Charter Marks website www.cabinetoffice.gov.uk/chartermark/.

Individuals (healthcare professionals and patients)

Healthcare professionals: The clinical governance framework provides infrastructures that facilitate the continued professional development of individuals, which should be aligned to contracts of employment, the KSF (DH 2004b), human resources policies and procedures that are all linked to the concept of lifelong learning. To support the integration of lifelong learning and the continued professional development of staff, supporting structures, such as the following, need to be in place to encourage this process:

- Organisational objectives
- Performance appraisal aligned to KSF (as outlined previously in this chapter)
- Personal development plans (PDPs)

- Principles of honesty and openness
- Access to education and training
- Access to adequate and appropriate resources
- Management support, e.g. whistle blowing policy and procedures
- Proactive rather than reactive approaches to untoward incidents or complaints
- The development of a learning organisation and culture

Patients: The public needs to be assured that they not only will receive the best quality service and care but also will be active partners directly involved in this provision. Where required, special groups or individuals will be involved in service evaluations and developments such as developing service for individuals with disability, e.g. deafness, learning disabilities. Patients should be actively encouraged to participate in and be regarded as equal partners in health service development, planning, implementation, delivery and evaluation of services. The Patient Advice and Liaison Services (PALS) and Patient and Public Involvement Forum (PPIF) Organisation (DH 2003) should be instrumental in facilitating and monitoring this process. The PPIFs are about to be replaced with Local Involvement Networks (LINKS) DH 2006b).

In summary, quality information is essential to achieve effective infrastructures for the implementation, monitoring and evaluation of the systems and processes associated with clinical governance. 'Good communication (information-giving and receiving) flow is fundamental to clinical governance and accountability' (O'Neill 2000, p. 816). Accountability is our final piece of the jigsaw in Fig. 3.3, which will now be explored in more detail in relation to clinical governance.

Accountability

Figure 3.3 illustrates how clinical governance is everybody's business, with all clinical and non-clinical staff responsible for ensuring that they are actively involved in managing and minimising clinical risks. This can only be accomplished if they have the necessary knowledge, understanding and skills to perform their roles efficiently and effectively. Continuous quality improvement is at the heart of all practices, which are regularly monitored with a view to improved performance based on a foundation of efficient and effective channels of communication and information-giving. In essence accountability can be defined as 'the requirement that each nurse (healthcare professional) is answerable and responsible for the outcome of his or her professional actions' (Pennels 1997).

Accountability within the context of clinical governance could be viewed at three levels – the organisation, team and individual – all having the responsibility for implementing, monitoring and evaluating the key components of clinical governance within their role. For example, the Trust board's chief executive is accountable to parliament in ensuring compliance of best clinical practice, which is founded on the principles of clinical governance. This can only be achieved and demonstrated by having robust systems of communication, risk management, performance management, quality improvement programmes and effective information systems. Likewise a team (ward/unit/department/GP surgery/General

---

Activity 3.1: Feedback: Key components of clinical governance

It is evident from the contents of this chapter that clinical governance is dependent on having an organisational culture that is open, honest and transparent in the way it deals with untoward incidents, complaints and accolades derived from internal or external sources, i.e. staff or the public. To foster this type of culture a managerial style that proactively encourages staff development and continuous learning is fundamental if an organisation aims to achieve continuous quality improvements. Quality improvements are the overriding aim of clinical governance, which is dependent on having the correct systems and processes in place to assure quality for the organisation, teams and individuals. The following systems and processes need to operate efficiently, effectively and harmoniously if clinical governance is to be successful at all these levels of a healthcare organisation:

- Risk management
- Performance management
- Quality improvement programmes
- Information
- Accountability.

Activity 3.2: Feedback: Performance management

It is evident from the section on performance management that several factors may have a positive or negative impact on an individual's, team's or organisation's performance, such as the following:

- Management
- Culture
- Environment
- Effective communication.

Issues surrounding either the individual's, team's or organisation's 'performance' are associated with the above factors, which are primarily communicated via two sources: the public's perceived experiences of a healthcare provision and the organisational evidence such as untoward incidents, clinical complaints and quality outcomes.

Dental Practitioner surgery) needs to have similar systems to demonstrate the delivery of best practice.

It is clear from Fig. 3.3 that if you base your practice on these key principles your accountability to the public, employer, patients and profession can only be enhanced along with the standard and quality of care offered. In light of the recent healthcare reforms and media interest in healthcare (Chapter 1), it is essential that you become familiar with what accountability truly means. 'Accountability is like pregnancy – you cannot be slightly pregnant and you cannot be slightly accountable' (Glover 1999). To be truly accountable and fit for practice we would suggest that you address the following questions:

- What are the contributing factors for change in individual and professional practice?
- What might be the consequences of not changing or developing professional practice?
- How can you ensure that your practice is evidence based?
- How do you know that your practice is efficient and effective?

You will then be equipped with the knowledge, understanding and skills to support your professional accountability. If you familiarise yourself with the issues contained within this chapter and adopt the principles of lifelong learning to address any subsequent gaps in your own knowledge and skills, you will be demonstrating your ability to justify clinical judgements relating to accountability, legal and professional issues and subsequent advances in your practice.

Conclusion

This chapter has outlined in detail the key components of clinical governance and their relationship to organisations, teams and individuals in the pursuit of clinical excellence. The challenges for many healthcare professionals are not in describing or explaining what clinical governance is, but in applying and working with this concept in their daily practice(s). Chapter 4 provides practical advice and guidance on how clinical governance could be implemented to support the organisation, teams and individuals. We would suggest that clinical governance will only become truly effective where the public are an integral part of the process. That is when the patients, carers and service users inform healthcare professionals and their employing organisations of when things go well or not so well. Service improvement, development and innovation can no longer be left in the hands of healthcare professionals alone.

Key points

- Clinical governance is about promoting and achieving continuous improvement within healthcare organisations and professional practice.
- Clinical excellence is dependent on having a proactive management and leadership style and honest and open culture.
- Innovations and good practices are shared and lessons learnt from not so good practices.
- Clinical governance is dependent on the unification, integration and harmonisation of six key systems and processes contained within a healthcare organisation:

  (1) Risk management
  (2) Performance management
  (3) Quality improvement
  (4) Information
  (5) Accountability
  (6) Communication.

- Lifelong learning, continuous professional development and the integration of evidence into practice through robust research and development infrastructures are of paramount importance in achieving quality improvements within the clinical governance frameworks.
- Patients, carers and service users should be viewed as integral and equal partners in service development, planning, implementation, delivery and evaluation.

Suggested reading

Baker, M. (1998) *Making Sense of the NHS White Papers*, 2nd edn. Radcliffe Medical Press, Oxford.

Department of Health (2000) *An organization with a memory*. Report of an expert group on learning from adverse incidents in the NHS chaired by the Chief Medical Officer. DH, London.

Mayatt, I.L. (2004) (ed) *Tolley's Managing Risk in Healthcare: Law and Practice*, 2nd edn. LexisNexis, Croyden.

Muir Gray, J.A. (1997) *Evidence-based Healthcare: How to Make Health Policy and Management Decisions*. Churchill Livingstone, London.

NHS Executive (1999) *Health Service Circular 1999/065 Clinical Governance: Quality in the New NHS*. DH, London.

NHS Executive (1999) *Health Service Circular 1999/154 Continuing Professional Development: Quality in the New NHS*. DH, London.

O'Neill, S. (2000) Clinical governance in action. Part 4: Communication. *Professional Nurse*, 16 (1) 816–817.

Pearce, P. & McSherry, R. (2000) Development: making it happen. *Healthcare Risk Report*, 6 (10) 15–17.

RCN (2000) *Clinical Governance: How Nurses Can Get Involved*. Royal College of Nursing, London.

Sealey, C. (1999) Clinical governance; an information guide for occupational therapists. *British Journal of Occupational Therapy*, 62 (6) 263–268.

Squire, S. & Cullen, R. (2001) Clinical governance in action. Part 7: Effective learning. *Professional Nurse*, 16 (4) 1014–1015.

Wilson, J. & Tingle, J. (eds) (1999) *Clinical Risk Modification: A Route to Clinical Governance*. Butterworth Heinemann, Oxford.

References

Audit Commission (1992) *What Seems to Be the Matter? Communication Between Hospitals and Patients*. Audit Commission, London.

Baker, M. (1998) *Making Sense of the NHS White Papers*, 2nd Edn. Radcliffe Medical Press, Oxford.

Collins, W. (1985) *The New Collins Concise Dictionary*. Guild Publishing Company, London.

Commission for Health Improvement Investigations (2004) *Lessons from CHI Investigation 2000–2003*. The Stationery Office, London.

Crombie, I.K. (1996) *The Pocket Guide to Critical Appraisal*. BMJ Publishing Group, London.

Cullum, N., DiCenso, A. & Ciliska, D. (1998) Implementing evidence based nursing; some misconceptions. *Evidence Based Medicine*, 1 (2) 38–40.

Department of Health (1992a) *The Patient's Charter; Raising the Standards*. The Stationery Office, London.

Department of Health (1992b) *The Citizen's Charter*. The Stationery Office, London.

Department of Health (1994) *Corporate Governance in the NHS, Code of Conduct, Code of Accountability*. The Stationery Office, London.

Department of Health (1997a) *The New NHS: Modern, Dependable*. DH, London.

Department of Health (1997b) *Code of Openness in the NHS*. The Stationery Office, London.

Department of Health (1998) *Quality in the New NHS*. DH, London.

Department of Health (2000a) *An organisation with a memory*. Report of an expert group on learning from adverse incidents in the NHS chaired by the Chief Medical Officer. DH, London.

Department of Health (2000b) *Improving Working Lives Standard*. DH, London.

Department of Health (2001) *Building a Safer NHS for Patients: Implementing an Organisation with a Memory*. DH, London.

Department of Health (2003) *Core National Standards and Evaluation Frameworks: Assessing Performance Against National Core Standards for PALS*.

DH, London. http://www.dh.gov.uk/PublicationsAndStatistics/Publications/
PublicationsPolicyAndGuidance/PublicationsPolicyAndGuidanceArticle/fs/en?
CONTENT_ID=4119314&chk=OCJDFT.

Department of Health (2004a) *Agenda for Change – What Will it Mean for You?
A Guide for Staff.* DH, London.

Department of Health (2004b) *The Knowledge and Skills Framework (NHSKSF)
and Development Review Process (October 2004).* DH, London.

Department of Health (2004c) *Standards for Better Health: Healthcare Standards
for Services Under the NHS – A Consultation Document.* DH, London.

Department of Health (2006a) *Update Our Health, Our Care, Our Say.* HMSO,
London. http://www.dh.gov.uk/assetRoot/04/12/76/28/04127628.pdf.

Department of Health (2006b) *A Stronger Voice: A Framework for Creating a
Stronger Local Voice in the Development of Health and Social Care Services.*
DH, London.

Donaldson, L.J. (2000) Clinical governance; a mission to improve. *British Journal
of Clinical Governance,* 5 (1) 6–7.

Donaldson, L.J. & Muir Gray, J.A. (1998) Clinical governance: a quality duty for
health organizations. *Quality in Healthcare,* 7 (Suppl.) S37–S44.

Edwards, J. & Packham, R. (1999) A model for the practical implementation of
clinical governance. *Journal of Clinical Excellence,* 1 (1) 13–18.

Garland, G. (1998) Governance. *Nursing Management,* 5 (6) 28–31.

Glacken, M. (2004) Perceived barriers and facilitators to implementing research findings in the Irish practice setting. *Journal of Clinical Nursing,* 136,
731/746.

Glover, D. (1999) *Accountability. Nursing Times Monograph.* Emap Healthcare,
London.

Kitson, A. (1997) Using evidence to demonstrate the values of nursing. *Nursing
Standard,* 11 (28) 34–39.

Long, A. & Harrison, S. (1996) Evidence based decision making. *Health Service
Journal,* 106, 11 January, 1–11.

Martin, V. (2000) How to manage, Part 6. Individual Performance. *Appraisal
Nursing Times,* 96 (21) 41.

May, A., Alexander, C. & Mulhall, A. (1998) Research utilization in nursing:
barriers and opportunities. *Journal of Clinical Effectiveness,* 32, 59–63.

Mayatt, V.L. (1995) *The CNST – how to meet the risk management standards
and reduce financial losses.* HRRI Conference, Edinburgh, Paper Sedgwick UK
Ltd.

Mayatt, V.L. (2004) (ed) *Tolley's Managing Risk in Healthcare: Law and
Practice,* 2nd edn. LexisNexis, Croyden.

McCabe, C. & Timmins, F. (2006) *Communication Skills for Nursing Practice.*
Palgrave Macmillan, Basingstoke.

McSherry, R. (2004) Practice development and healthcare governance: a recipe
for modernisation. *Journal of Nursing Management,* 12, 137–146.

McSherry, R. & Haddock, J. (1999) Evidence based healthcare: its place within
clinical governance. *British Journal of Nursing,* 8 (2) 113–117.

McSherry, R., Simmons, M. & Abbott, P. (2001) *Evidence Informed Nursing: A
Guide for Clinical Nurses.* Routledge, London.

McSherry, R., Artley, A. & Holloran, J. (2006) Research awareness: an important factor for evidence based nursing. *World Views on Evidence Based Nursing* (in press).

National Audit Office (2005) *A Safer Place for Patients: Learning to Improve Patients' Safety.* NAO, London. http://www.nao.org.uk/publications/nao_reports/05-06/0506456.pdf.

National Patient Safety Agency (2003a) *Patient Safety Alert.* 23 July. NPSA, London.

National Patient Safety Agency (2003b) *Introduction to the National Reporting and Learning System.* http://www.npsa.nhs.uk/public/reporting/intoduction.

National Patient Safety Agency (2004) *Patient Safety Alert 02. Establishing a Standard Crash Telephone Number in Hospitals.* NPSA, London.

NHS Executive (1999a) *Health Service Circular 1999/065 Clinical Governance: Quality in the New NHS.* DH, London.

NHS Executive (1999b) *Health Services Circular 1999/154 Continuing Professional Development: Quality in the New NHS.* DH, London.

NHS Executive (1999c) *Health Service Circular 1999/053 for the Record: Managing Records in NHS Trusts and Health Authorities.* DH, London.

NHS Executive (2000a) *Information for Health.* DH, London.

NHS Executive (2000b) *Health Service Circular 2000/Caldicott Report.* DH, London.

National Health Service Litigation Authority (2006) *Welcome to the National Health Service Litigation Authority.* NHSLA, London. http://www.nhsla.com/.

O'Neill, S. (2000) Clinical governance in action. Part 4: Communication. *Professional Nurse,* 16 (1) 816–817.

Pallen, N. & Timmins, F. (2002) Research based practice: myth or reality. A review of the barriers affecting research utilisation. *Nurse Education in Practice,* 2 (2) 99–108.

Pearce, P. & McSherry, R. (2000) Development: making it happen. *Healthcare Risk Report,* 6 (10) 15–17.

Pennels, C. (1997) Nursing and the law: clinical responsibility. *Professional Nurse,* 13 (3) 162–164.

RCN (2000) *Clinical Governance: How Nurses Can Get Involved.* Royal College of Nursing, London.

Rycroft-Malone, J., Harvey, G., Seers, K., Kitson, A., McCormack, B. & Titchen, A. (2004) An exploration of the factors that influence the implementation of evidence into practice. *Journal of Clinical Nursing,* 13 (8) 913–924.

Sackett, L.D., Rosenburg, W. & Haynes, B.R. (1997) *Evidence Based Medicine; How to Practise and Teach EBM.* Churchill Livingstone, London.

Scally, G. & Donaldson, L.J. (1998) Clinical governance and the drive for quality improvement in the new NHS in England. *BMJ,* 137, 61–65.

Swage, T. (1998) Clinical care takes center stage. *Nursing Times,* 94 (14) 40–41.

Walshe, K., Freeman, T., Latham, L., Wallace, P. & Spurgeon, P. (2000) *Clinical Governance: From Policy to Practice.* Health Services Management Centre, University of Birmingham.

West, M.A., Borrill, C., Dawson, J., Scully, J., Carter, M., Anelay, A., Patterson, M. & Waring, J. (2000) The link between the management of employees and patient mortality in acute hospitals. *International Journal of Human Resource Management*, 138.

Williams, C.A. & Heins, R.M. (1976) *Risk Management and Insurance*. McGraw-Hill, New York.

Wilson, J. & Tingle, J. (eds) (1999) *Clinical Risk Modification: A Route to Clinical Governance*. Butterworth Heinemann, Oxford.

Chapter 4

Applying Clinical Governance in Daily Practice

Rob McSherry and Paddy Pearce

Introduction

Chapter 3 explored in detail the key components of clinical governance and the systems and processes necessary for its success. This chapter builds on the previous chapters by offering practical examples on how to facilitate the application of the clinical governance framework at an organisational, team and individual level. To make the introduction of clinical governance easier it is important that any organisation, team or individual is clear about what clinical governance is and why it is important to the promotion of clinical quality (Chapter 2).

Clinical governance is 'a framework through which NHS organisations are accountable for continuously improving the quality of their services and safeguarding high standards of care, by creating an environment in which clinical excellence in clinical care will flourish' (DH 1997). It emerges from this definition that the successful development, implementation and evaluation of clinical governance frameworks is associated with 'two distinct elements – the mechanistic element of ensuring systems are in place, and the more philosophical element of producing a culture in which clinical quality can flourish' (Haslock 1999, p. 744).

To advance clinical governance within the NHS, all healthcare organisations need to establish their level of quality as required by the Department of Health in the Health Service Circular HSC 1999/065 (NHS Executive 1999). To achieve these standards within any healthcare organisation a baseline assessment of the organisation's existing systems and processes is required. The baseline assessment is necessary to reveal strengths and weaknesses of existing systems and processes so that a robust action plan can be developed to facilitate the development, implementation and evaluation of clinical governance. The baseline assessment should be linked to the Standards for Better Health (DH 2004) or other relevant agencies' standards, e.g. the Commission for Social Care Inspection (CSCI). The difficulty for many healthcare organisations, teams and individuals is, where does this process begin? We would suggest that for the newly configured PCTs commencing in October 2006, it would be prudent to conduct a baseline assessment.

Introducing clinical governance into healthcare organisations

Given the importance that the government attaches to clinical governance, by making the healthcare organisations' chief executives accountable for the successful implementation of clinical governance structures in the pursuit of clinical excellence, it is easy to see why many of the leads for clinical governance are members of the executive board, i.e. Medical Directors or Directors of Nursing. The rationale for this is quite simple: clinical governance is about achieving high quality within clinical and non-clinical services. Therefore it is important that any strategy is led by a clinician who has the respect and confidence of his or her peers, along with an ability to influence, guide and lead fellow healthcare professionals through the change management process.

For all healthcare organisations the first step towards implementing clinical governance is the identification of individuals to be given the lead responsibility for taking forward the development, implementation and evaluation of a clinical governance strategy. Having identified the lead person responsible for the strategic development of the clinical governance framework, clinical governance committees (CGCs), healthcare governance committee (HCG) and/or integrated governance committees (IGC) have been developed as subcommittees of healthcare organisations' executive boards. The CGC, HCG or IGC comprise of senior members of staff representing various professional, human resources and managerial aspects of the organisation, with an overview of and responsibility for maintaining key components of the clinical governance framework, i.e. clinical risk, quality, performance management and professional development, as illustrated in Fig. 4.1.

Figure 4.1 describes the hierarchical relationships between the management levels, professional groups and the key components of clinical governance. Each tier of the triangle is responsible for its own practice and accountable to the next tier, for example the clinical governance subcommittee is accountable and reports to the Trust board. Examples of how clinical governance has been introduced into various healthcare organisations are offered by Edwards and Packham (1999), Haslock (1999) and Starke and Boden (1999).

The CGC's initial task was to ensure that a baseline assessment of its organisation's capability and capacity to implement clinical governance was performed in accordance with the guidance issued with the HSC 1999/065. Today we would argue that the CGC, HCG or IGC are

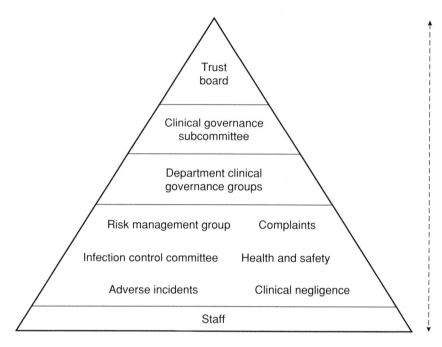

The dashed line illustrates how effective clinical governance is
dependent on two-way channels of communication

Fig. 4.1   Management structure associated with clinical governance.

responsible for undertaking the baseline and for approving, implementing
and monitoring the effectiveness of healthcare governance subsequent to
a development plan resulting from the baseline. So what does baseline
assessment and development look like?

Clinical governance: what is a baseline assessment and development plan?

The HSC 1999/065 guidance provides in annex 2 a matrix of the standards requiring action by NHS Trusts, Health Authorities, Primary Care
Groups and Primary Care Trusts. These standards needed to be agreed
with the NHS Executive regional offices, indicating how the key components of clinical governance were to be achieved for their respective organisations. A critical review of annex 2 reveals the main components of what
a baseline assessment should consist of in demonstrating whether the organisation has the capability and capacity to deliver clinical governance. The
annex can be summarised into four key areas, as illustrated in Box 4.1.

The questions raised in Box 4.1 are synonymous with the information
presented in Fig. 3.3 – the key components of clinical governance which

> **Box 4.1 Components of clinical governance baseline assessments**
>
> - Does your organisation have clear lines of accountability for the overall quality of clinical care and can this be demonstrated?
> - Are there comprehensive systems for continuous quality improvement at all levels of the organisation?
> - Is there a strategy for risk management and risk reductions?
> - Does the organisation have an operational system for clinical performance management?
> - Are there robust efficient and effective information systems for the collection and dissemination of information to influence practice.

describe in detail the systems and processes necessary for the successful development, implementation and evaluation of clinical governance. Figure 3.3 offers a framework that if used could provide organisations, teams and individuals with useful information regarding the initial clinical governance status and subsequent evaluations.

Table 4.1 offers a checklist for undertaking a baseline assessment of clinical governance based on the information obtained from HSC 1999/065 (Lim *et al.* 2000).

From the information obtained from the baseline assessment shown in Table 4.1, an in-depth action plan should be formulated building upon the strengths and weaknesses identified by the baseline assessment in measuring progress in advancing clinical governance in the areas of 'performance, developing infrastructures, staff and board development, planning and prioritisation' (NHS Executive 1999, p. 2). Essentially the action plan developed from the baseline assessment should have realistic expectations in relation to:

- Aims and objectives
- Goals
- Actions
- Time-scales
- Responsible individual(s)

These expectations should be shared with all levels of staff. Having shared this information with staff, directorates, wards or departments, they need to conduct their own local baseline assessment and formulate an action plan to achieve their specific and overall actions identified by the organisational baseline assessment (RCN 1998). This approach nurtures the philosophy embedded in the concept of clinical governance by involving all staff from the outset in creating an environment in which clinical excellence can flourish. The application of this approach reaffirms the notion that the outcome of the baseline assessment is a true reflection and

Table 4.1 Baseline assessment checklist.

Standards	Full compliance	Partial compliance	Non-compliance	Additional comments
Risk management Risk management strategy and policies associated with clinical and non-clinical aspects of service		✓		
Compliance with CNST standards	✓			Level 2 CNST
Systems for reporting and detecting: equipment failure		✓		
Managing performance Systems for reporting and detecting: ● Complaints ● Clinical incidents ● Untoward incidents ● Individual performance review	✓ ✓ ✓ ✓			Consultant IPR introduced April 2001

Quality improvement				
Clinical audit	✓			
Compliance with NICE and NSFs guidelines/recommendations		✓		
Evidence-based practice		✓		
Continuing professional development		✓		
Quality information				
Clinical information systems		✓		
Clinical outcomes data		✓		
Comparative data		✓		
Benchmarking			✓	
Accountability				
Policies and procedures	✓			All policies and procedures to be reviewed annually
Regular reporting to boards on efficiency and effectiveness of clinical governance		✓		Monthly reports to boards

NB: Reference should be made to *Standards for Better Health* (DH 2004) when completing this table.

representation of the organisational, team and individual levels, making future strategies for change easier to manage because clinical governance is everybody's business – a view echoed in the following statement:

'If clinical governance becomes some sort of parallel universe detached from day to day management and practice, it is likely to produce a resented bureaucracy that fails to deliver. It is only by embedding its principles and practice into everyday care delivery and organisation that it will succeed.' (Haslock 1999, p. 747)

To ensure that clinical governance does not become a bureaucratic 'nightmare' as alluded to by Haslock, staff must be fully informed of the managerial and strategic direction for the development, implementation and monitoring of clinical governance within the organisation, as outlined in Fig. 4.1. This could be done by having clinical governance briefing sessions, newsletters and governance seminars, and learning and sharing from incidents which ideally involve staff in the early stages of the process. Activity 4.1 will assist you in ascertaining whether your organisation is successful.

Activity 4.1: Clinical governance: baseline assessment questions

During the early stages of a clinical governance baseline assessment it is essential that staff can correctly answer the following questions in order to act as a starting point for the development of clinical governance:

- Who leads clinical governance in your organisation?
- Is there a manager responsible for clinical governance?
- Who is the clinical governance lead for your directorate, team and department?
- Is there a clinical governance lead for your professional group within your organisation?
- Have you been involved with the baseline assessment at either organisational, team or individual level?
- Have you had any awareness training on clinical governance and how it may affect you and what you do?

Feedback is provided at the end of the chapter.

Activity 4.1 is aimed at making you aware of how successfully your organisation's CGC, HCG or IGC communicated what and how clinical governance was to be implemented throughout your organisation. This stage in the process of developing clinical governance is essential in informing and involving staff before commencing the baseline assessment and subsequent development plan. Without staff's involvement in this process they are unlikely to understand and appreciate the importance of clinical governance at the clinical level; it will be seen to be owned purely by the senior management within the organisation. The clinical work-force may view this as yet another demand from government, construing it as not relevant to themselves or in the provision of services to patients. These misconceptions about clinical governance need to be tackled before and during the baseline assessment. Failure to follow this approach could be the reasons why clinical governance in some healthcare organisations is not owned and viewed positively by the clinical and non-clinical staff in everyday practice – a perception confirmed by the following comment

> 'much of the machinery of clinical governance at an NHS Trust [and Primary Care Trust] level is now in place. However, it seems that clin-ical governance has yet to make a real difference at the clinical workface, and that changes in culture which it demands of healthcare organisations have not really begun to happen yet.' (Walshe *et al.* 2000, p. 3)

The Walshe *et al.* (2000) statement was correct at the time. In 2006 it is possible to begin to highlight the impacts of clinical governance, which are detailed in Chapter 7. Following the development of a managerial and strategic framework for the development, implementation and monitor-ing of clinical governance, as illustrated in Fig. 4.1, and the informing of staff about this framework and subsequent implementation of the clinical governance baseline assessment, the next step is the writing and develop-ing of the clinical governance action plan. The aim of the action plan is eloquently articulated by the RCN in suggesting that the:

> 'Development plan shows how your organisation intends to build on what is working well, how it plans to improve, what it is doing less well and how it aims to fill any gaps.' (RCN 2000, p. 7)

What does a clinical governance action plan look like and why is it necessary?

The clinical governance action plan should be developed in light of the findings of the baseline assessment undertaken by the CGC, HCG or IGC or nominated representatives. A format of how an action plan could be presented is offered by Garland (1998), RCN (1998) and Sealey (1999). The baseline assessment should highlight the strengths and weaknesses of the organisation in achieving the standards outlined in Fig. 4.1. The action plan should contain realistic targets directed towards improving infrastructures, performance and quality at organisational, team and indi-vidual levels. In some healthcare professions, action plans are viewed negatively because they have predominantly been associated with poor performance and practices. In this instance clinical governance action plans should be viewed positively and used as a guide for continuous quality improvements and in the sharing of good practices and performances.

Appendix 4.1 provides a detailed template of a clinical governance development plan (for a local Primary Care Trust) broadly based on the key components associated with the clinical governance framework as highlighted in Fig. 3.3. The template provides a clinical governance assessment framework and development offering realistic aims and objectives, and identifies lead personnel to take responsibility within given time-scales for achieving each specific objective. The difficulty for some organisations, teams and individuals is relating the principles of clinical governance to their own specific daily practices (Malbon *et al.* 1998). Box 4.2 provides examples of case studies provided by other authors. The remainder of this chapter will use case studies taken from the authors' own experiences to demonstrate how clinical governance can be applied to our daily practices at an organisational, team and individual level.

Box 4.2

For examples of case studies relating to how clinical governance can be applied to clinical practice read:

Elcoat, C. (2000) Clinical governance in action: part 1. Key issues in clinical effectiveness. *Professional Nurse*, 15 (10) 622–623.
Kausar, S.A., Rowe, M. & Carr, J. (2000) Avoiding medication errors and adverse incident: the way forward. *Clinical Governance Bulletin*, 1 (2) 4–5.
Northcott, N. (1999) Clinical governance no. 1: organizational effectiveness – 1. *Nursing Times Learning Curves*, 3 (2) 10.

Case study 1: Applying the principles of clinical governance to an organisation

A local hospital Trust has received a number of complaints from patients, and their carers, who have recently been admitted and discharged from the acute medical wards following a stroke (cerebral vascular accident). The complaints could be classified under the headings of poor quality care and poor communication.

Poor quality care

- Patients not having their privacy and hygiene needs attended to
- Development of hospital-acquired pressure sores

- Failure to attend to nutritional needs
- Limited physiotherapy
- Delay in home assessment and discharge

Poor communication

- Limited information about the patient's illness from medical staff
- Inconsistent information from the professional staff
- Failure to disclose information about patients' falls

If each of these individual aspects of a complaint were reviewed in isolation it would be difficult to establish the severity of the problems associated with caring for stroke patients within this organisation. Having a clinical governance framework in operation within an organisation enables it to establish, understand and respond to clinical problems that are distressing to patients, carers and staff – a point echoed by Garside (1999):

> 'the big opportunity offered by clinical governance is the opportunity to change systems – to pull together different components and strands from the clinical and managerial worlds to improve things for patients.'

In light of this statement let us explore in detail how the systems and processes associated with clinical governance apply to the case study as illustrated in Fig. 4.2.

Figure 4.2 illustrates how the key components of clinical governance can be applied and demonstrated in action at the organisation level. The case study demonstrates how clinical governance offers continuous quality improvement by working in collaboration with the various departments and their associated systems and processes (Northcott 1999).

In this instance when the complaints had been investigated the main issues were about poor quality not related to individual clinicians but to the systems and processes that clinicians had to work in. An analysis of the complaints revealed two areas within the clinical governance framework that required urgent attention: poor quality and poor communication, particularly information gathering and disseminating. The application of the clinical governance framework to this situation enabled a full review of the current standards of practices and this was subsequently reviewed against the best available evidence, and recommendations made and implemented in light of the findings.

The overall outcome of this case study reinforces the need for reviewing untoward incidents or failures that have a recurring theme or pattern at an organisational level based upon a systems and processes approach, rather than at an individual level. The outcome of the clinical audit based

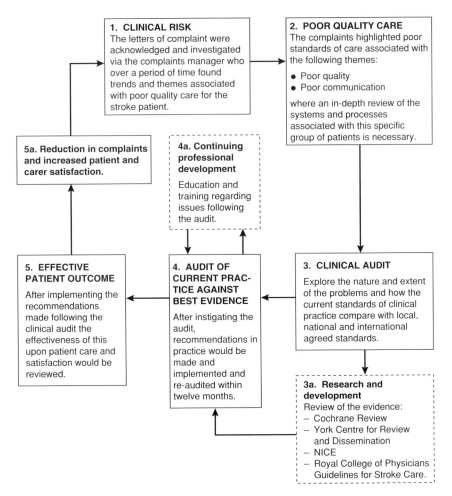

Fig. 4.2　Applying the principles of clinical governance at organisational level.

on the application of the best available evidence could make strong recommendations for the following:

- The need for a continuing professional development programme because the findings of the audit could have revealed a deficit in the clinical and management's knowledge with regard to best practices for stroke patients'/carers' care.
- The provision of a specialist stroke unit or designated rehabilitation area where patients receive high quality multidisciplinary care from specialist healthcare professions.

These points are more likely to be addressed as the recommendations are based on a thorough review of the current service provision using the clinical governance framework. A framework applied in this instance highlighted clinical risks, poor quality, and ineffective communications and information-giving which, if not attended to, could lead to increased levels of complaints and loss of local public confidence in this healthcare organisation. The long-term impact of this poor quality service could culminate in low staff morale and subsequent high levels of sickness and absence, thus exacerbating this clinical situation. As this statement describes: a poor lead organisation with a closed culture equals a clinical disaster waiting to happen. In this instance the notion of accountability becomes everyone's business.

The principles behind this case study could equally be applied to evaluating the existing practices for teams and departments within Acute Trusts, Primary Care Trusts, the Mental Health Trust, Ambulance Trust and in the Independent Healthcare Sector. The emphasis is on disseminating good or not so good practice – a point reinforced by Smith (1998) when describing the effects of the Bristol Case (see Chapter 1) where poor practices, performances and a closed culture culminated in higher than expected mortality rates for children undergoing cardiac surgery; and similarly to the findings of the Rowan Ward (a mental health unit located in the North West of England) enquiry by the Commission for Health Improvement (2003). In the later cases the HC also noted that the local PCT had failed to assure themselves of the quality of a commissioned service.

Case study 2: Applying the principles of clinical governance to a team

Case study 1 highlighted how the clinical governance framework can be applied to the organisation-wide situation in addressing poor practice and performance. Case study 2 explores how clinical governance can be used in a positive way to assist clinical teams to improve the services they provide.

An orthopaedic ward in a District General Hospital with a large elderly population had a higher than expected incidence of fractured hips (fractured neck of femur). This demand on the emergency services led to increased waiting times for elective orthopaedic surgery such as total hip and knee replacements. The situation was further exacerbated by the shortage of qualified nursing staff within the orthopaedic specialty to care for this specific client group along with a shortage of Physiotherapists and Occupational Therapists to provide rehabilitative support. In this instance no reported clinical complaints were recorded via the incident reporting systems or the complaints procedures. Clinical governance was used in a proactive way to support the healthcare professionals, managers and patients in developing new ways of improving the service and in responding to staff's concerns of not meeting government waiting list targets for elective surgery. Furthermore, the issues associated with low morale resulting from a perceived provision of suboptimal care were addressed. Figure 4.3 illustrates the systems and processes associated with the application of a clinical governance framework to support a service improvement at team level.

Figure 4.3 shows how the clinical governance framework can be used to enhance the quality of a service at team level by the harmonising of the various key components associated with clinical governance. We acknowledge that waiting times for elective surgery have improved significantly (Pearce & McSherry 2006); however, this remains an issue in certain specialities where there is a shortage of healthcare specialists (Boseley 2002). In this instance a *performance management issue* was detected via the feedback from regional offices, stating that the Trust's targets for elective orthopaedic surgery were not being achieved. Yet, the principle behind the case study could be applied to resolve other performance management related issues. A *quality issue* was evident from several points of view:

- The quality of life of elderly patients and their families is deteriorating while the patients are on a long waiting list
- Patients are older and sicker when they are eventually admitted
- Hospital length of stay is increased
- Waiting lists become longer
- Services become more expensive and quality is impaired
- Healthcare professionals become demoralised as a consequence of not providing the service to a level they would like to

In light of the above performance and quality issues an *organisational audit* of the orthopaedics multidisciplinary teams was conducted to see where improvements in the current service provisions could be made. *The review process* required all staff to be involved so that local ownership and participation in the development of the new services were agreed by all members of the multidisciplinary teams. This proactive collaborative approach to continuous quality improvement is vital for the success or failure of any change – a challenge that is perhaps difficult and sometimes viewed as being unrealistic in today's NHS (Northcott 1999). The review process requires staff involvement in both accessing and reviewing best practices in the development and application of the new methods employed in resolving this clinical situation. To resolve the issues identified within this case study an integrated care pathway was developed and introduced after communication with and collaboration and education of

Fig. 4.3 Service improvements facilitated by the application of a clinical governance framework at team level.

all the staff to ensure the most efficient and effective reallocation of resources.

In this case study, 48 hours after surgical intervention the patients are nursed on an elderly rehabilitation ward with the appropriate staffing levels to assist with the rehabilitation process. An integrated care pathway was instigated in this instance to 'ensure multidisciplinary processes of patient focused care which specify key events, tests and assessments occurring in timely fashion to produce the best prescribed outcomes, within the resources and activities, for an appropriate episode of care' (Clinical Negligence Scheme for Trusts 1996). The integrated care pathway would ensure that an auditable trail of the patient's journey could be obtained and reviewed because 'the expected outcomes, frequently specified at different stages of the care pathway, are clearly described and any deviation or failure to achieve these outcomes or interim goals is quickly identified' (Benton 2000, p. 97). The drawback of this approach to providing care is that it can be viewed as cook-book healthcare.

The culmination of this approach ensures that the amount of orthopaedic elective surgery is increased because the beds are utilised more effectively. Failure by the clinical team to address this issue in a proactive way with the support of management and the clinical and non-clinical staff could eventually lead to increased patients' complaints or untoward incidents, making the need for change a reactive not proactive one – an approach that would certainly have an impact on the healthcare professionals working within this specialty area.

Essentially case study 2 demonstrates how using a proactive approach to implementing clinical governance can bring about improvements for patients, staff and management by the use of multidisciplinary collaboration partnerships in creating an environment and culture where all parties are involved from the outset.

As the saying goes, 'a problem shared is a problem halved'. How can we afford not to adopt this type of approach to promote continuous quality improvement?

The final case study in highlighting how clinical governance can be applied to the clinical situation focuses on its relevance to the individual healthcare professional.

Case study 3: Systems and processes associated with the application of a clinical governance framework at an individual level

Case study 3 is adapted from the second case study in an article by McSherry (1999) in *Health Care Risk Report* that explored the value of practice and professional development in assisting an organisation and individual to use the principles of clinical governance in daily practice.

A 38-year-old woman complains to her local hospital on discharge. Following her admission on to the acute medical ward for treatment of painful joints, she says a senior healthcare professional (could be a nurse, doctor or any healthcare professional who undertakes adjustments to extend or expand their roles) was abrupt and insensitive when inserting a cannula into her right hand. This caused unnecessary bruising and discomfort because the person concerned tried several times to insert the cannula without success. The woman stated that it was not until a more experienced member of staff saw what was happening and took over this duty from the staff member that the cannula was inserted on the first attempt.

Let us explore in detail how clinical governance may assist in overcoming this clinical incident associated with an individual's practice. In recent years a nurse manager, on receiving this complaint, might have rushed into establishing how this had occurred and who was responsible for such an incident so that disciplinary procedures could be instigated. This reactionary approach to management does not bode well in the context of clinical governance that promotes a fair blame culture by the use of a proactive management style, as outlined in Chapter 3. Figure 4.4 illustrates how the key components of clinical governance can be applied to encourage the individual, team and organisation to learn and develop from this clinical incident.

In this case study the incident was reported via the clinical incident reporting system and was passed to the respective clinical manager for this directorate/ward to investigate and feedback the findings to the clinical risk management team for a response to be given to the client. To address and alleviate the situation the manager would discuss the incident with the individual and undertake a SWOT analysis of the individual's strengths, weaknesses, opportunities and threats. This would pay particular

Fig. 4.4 How the key components of clinical governance can be applied to an individual.

attention to the incident and ensure that the healthcare professional had the necessary knowledge, skills and competence to perform the role of venous cannulation. If it was established that he/she lacked the competency or capability then a personal development plan (PDP) would be jointly agreed and written. This would incorporate regular monthly evaluations with the line manager. The plan could cover education and training in cannulation, shadowing staff and encouraging professional development in clinical information and skills.

The period for the PDP would vary according to the individual's needs. The professional may have been unaware of the discomfort caused to the patient for many reasons – pressure of work, not enough knowledge or training, incompetence, etc. The development and implementation of a PDP could be seen as an important tool to promote quality and standards of patient care and of effective clinical risk management for the following reasons:

- A clinical incident was reported (patient complaint) and investigated
- An assessment of the individual's performance was undertaken (knowledge, skills and competency) against established research evidence
- A personal development plan was written, implemented and evaluated under supervision
- The overall outcome for patient and staff should be improved standards and quality of care
- Where possible the organisation should learn a lesson from this case to avoid recurrence

An example of a PDP can be found in Appendix 4.2. In addition to supporting the individual to resolve the issues surrounding poor practices and performance, a team or organisation could learn from this incident by reviewing their own practices and associated systems and processes aligned to the practising of intravenous cannulation. Case study 3 reinforces the concept of clinical governance at an individual level. It shows how practice and professional development can be enhanced under the key areas of clinical risk, performance management and quality improvement.

Summary of the case studies

The case studies offer practical examples of how clinical governance can be applied to an organisation, team and individuals in the pursuit of clinical excellence. Case study 1 demonstrates how complaints about poor quality care can be a driver for continuous quality improvements at an organisational level. Complaints that are predominantly viewed negatively enabled a positive outcome to be achieved for the organisation by exploring and linking the key components of clinical governance. Case study 2 illustrates the determination of staff to improve their clinical services at a team level by collaborative working and partnerships, redesigning a new clinical service for the care of a specific group of patients and for healthcare professionals. This culminated in the development of an integrated care pathway for patients with a hip fracture, thus enabling more efficient and effective use of services and thereby improving the overall performance and management of the organisation. Case study 3 highlights how a proactive approach to the poor performance of an individual can be seen as a learning experience to themselves, clinical teams and the organisation. In totality, the case studies demonstrate the clinical governance challenges in exploring how the principles can be applied across organisational boundaries (and sectoral frontiers) to ensure the overall management of the care pathway, as opposed to the organisational management of the episode of care.

Conclusion

In conclusion, this chapter has outlined how healthcare organisations' capabilities and capacities to introduce clinical governance were initially assessed and developed by means of a baseline assessment and clinical governance development plans. The difficulties for some organisations, teams and individuals is in transporting the findings of either the organisational or local development plans into clinical practice. To assist healthcare professionals to overcome this concern, three practice-based case studies were presented and reviewed in relation to how clinical governance can be applied to these unique situations. The case studies systematically related how and where the key components of clinical governance could be linked to the various systems and processes of a healthcare organisation or Trust. Practical advice and guidance were offered throughout the case studies to enable the reader to apply the key components of clinical governance to the organisation, team and individual level.

Several themes emerge following the application of the clinical governance framework and the associated key components to case studies, which have the potential to inhibit or enhance the uptake of the goal of clinical governance and thus promote continuous quality improvements and clinical excellence. Effective communication, collaboration and working in partnerships, and the development of a culture that values 'people' and their individual contribution to healthcare are essential if clinical governance is to be realised in the reforming agenda of the NHS. We would argue that it is not the organisational structures alone that create a quality organisation, service or team; it is the aspirations, vision and values of the people who work within and for the organisation.

> **Activity 4.1: Feedback: Clinical governance: baseline assessment questions**
>
> The initial stages of a baseline assessment should be concerned with ensuring that all staff can answer the questions in order to establish what is known and not known about the systems and processes associated with clinical governance within the organisation.
>
> If you are unable to answer these questions we suggest that you require education and training on how clinical governance is being developed within your own organisation.

Key points

- Individual healthcare professionals should familiarise themselves with their local clinical governance arrangements and infrastructures for delivering the clinical governance agenda in their respective organisation.
- All healthcare organisations should have a baseline assessment and clinical governance development plan to develop, monitor and evaluate the value of clinical governance to their own organisation.
- Clinical governance and its associated key components can be applied to three levels: the organisation, team and individuals.
- Clinical governance is everybody's business.
- A proactive management style and honest and open culture that values all staff, in seeking to learn from its mistakes in a fair blame culture, is well on the road to successfully achieving the clinical governance agenda.

Suggested reading

Edwards, J. & Packham, R. (1999) A model for the practical implementation of clinical governance. *Journal of Clinical Excellence*, 1 (1) 13–18.

McSherry, R. & Pearce, P. (2004) Healthcare standards: a critique of the Department of Health's national standards for the NHS. *Health Care Risk Report*, 10, 8 July/Aug.

RCN (2000) *Clinical Governance: How Nurses Can Get Involved*. Royal College of Nursing, London.

Sealey, C. (1999) Clinical governance: an information guide for occupational therapists. *British Journal of Occupational Therapy*, 62 (6) 263–268.

References

Benton, D.C. (2000) Clinical effectiveness. In: *Achieving Evidence-based Practice: A Handbook for Practitioners* (eds S. Hamer & G. Collinson). Baillière Tindall, London.

Boseley, S. (2002) New Ideas hampered by shortage of specialist staff. *The Guardian*, 5 August.

Commission for Health Improvement (2003) *Investigation in Matters Arising from Care on Rowan Ward, Manchester Mental Health and Social Care Trust.* CHI, London.

Clinical Negligence Scheme for Trusts (1996) *Risk Management Standards and Procedures; Manual of Guidance.* CNST, Bristol.

Department of Health (1997) *The New NHS: Modern, Dependable.* DH, London.

Department of Health (2004) *Standards for Better Health: Healthcare Standards for Services Under the NHS – A Consultation Document.* DH, London.

Edwards, J. & Packham, R. (1999) A model for the practical implementation of clinical governance. *Journal of Clinical Excellence*, 1 (1) 13–18.

Garland, G. (1998) Governance. *Nursing Management*, 5 (6) 28–31.

Garside, P. (1999) Book review. *Clinical Governance: Making it Happen* (eds M. Lugon & J. Secker-Walker). RSM Press, London. BMJ, 318, 881.

Haslock, I. (1999) Introducing clinical governance in an acute trust. *Hospital Medicine*, 60 (10) 744–747.

Lim, J., Burton, T. & Bowens, A. (2000) *What Elements Should Be Covered in a Clinical Governance Development Plan?* Nuffield Institute for Health, University of Leeds, and NHS Executive Northern & Yorkshire.

Malbon, G., Gillam, S. & Maysn, N. (1998) Onus points. *Health Services Journal*, 19, 28–29.

McSherry, R. (1999) Practice and professional development. *Health Care Risk Report*, 6 (1) 21–22.

McSherry, R. & Haddock, J. (1999) Evidence based health care: its place within clinical governance. *British Journal of Nursing*, 8 (2) 113–117.

NHS Executive (1999) *Health Service Circular 1999/065 Clinical Governance: Quality in the New NHS.* DH, London.

Northcott, N. (1999) Clinical governance. Effective staff – 2. *Nursing Times*, 3 (4) 10.

Pearce, P. & McSherry, R. (2006) From stars to health checks: looking towards the future. *Health Care Risk Report* 12 (3) 12–14.

RCN (1998) *Guidance for Nurses on Clinical Governance.* Royal College of Nursing, London.

RCN (2000) *Clinical Governance: How Nurses Can Get Involved.* Royal College of Nursing, London.

Sealey, C. (1999) Clinical governance: an information guide for occupational therapists. *British Journal of Occupational Therapy*, 62 (6) 263–268.

Smith, R. (1998) All changed, changed utterly; British medicine will be transformed by the Bristol Case. *BMJ*, 316, 1917–1918.

Starke, D. & Boden, L. (1999) Case study – how to make it work. *Health Care Risk Report*, 6 (1) 18–20.

Walshe, K., Freeman, T., Latham, L., Wallace, L. & Spurgeon, P. (2000) *Clinical Governance: From Policy to Practice*. University of Birmingham.

Appendix 4.1
An example of a clinical governance action plan

As discussed earlier in this chapter, the clinical governance committee would establish the strategic direction for reviewing the status of the Trust's capability and capacity to achieve the standards outlined in annex 2 of the Health Service Circular 1999/065. Since the publication of the Health Service Circular 1999/065 many organisations have ongoing development plans to continuously improve the governance of their organisation. To comply with these standards a local baseline assessment would be performed by nominated parties where a development plan was formulated outlining areas of good and not so good compliance. This process is ongoing. Following the formulation of the development plan the organisation should decide the best way to implement, monitor and evaluate the development plan. To do this successfully clinical directorates or departments need to develop clinical governance implementation groups or committees that are multidisciplinary, containing members from each of the main departments of the Trust, as well as key personnel such as clinical risk managers, governance managers and other relevant parties. The clinical governance implementation group's responsibility is to oversee the development plan for its respective area by prioritising the work and producing a detailed project implementation plan for its completion. Below is an example of a written development plan that could support the organisation and directorate in achieving the standards outlined in HSC 1999/065.

To identify gaps in the present performance of the organisation and to bring these departments up to the desired standard the aims of the development plan could be as follows:

- To ensure all clinicians are involved in relevant evidence audit programmes.
- To ensure full participation in relevant national confidential inquiries, e.g. confidential enquiry into perioperative deaths (CEPOD).
- To ensure that the clinical standards of the national service frameworks (NSFs) and National Institute for Health and Clinical Excellence (NICE) recommendations are implemented.
- To ensure that the clinical audit programme reflects the organisation's clinical governance agenda.
- To enhance risk management and performance systems and processes.
- To promote continued professional development of staff.

Clinical governance development plan, 2003 onwards

Section 1: The patient's experience

STRENGTHS	WEAKNESSES

• Well developed systems of user involvement in Mental Health
  ○ Multidisciplinary service governance group
  ○ Regular patient satisfaction surveys
• Patient involvement in CHD LIT group and Diabetes review group
• PALS has been established
• PCT Patient Forum has been established
• Began the process of developing the Patient and Public Involvement (PPI) PCT policy and established a group to progress this agenda
• Experienced and skilled staff
• Regular patient satisfaction surveys carried out in Community Dental Services
• Good results from CHI National Patient Survey
• Few patient complaints
• High levels of public interest
• Lots of good practice inherited from predecessor organisations
• Received focus award from DOH/BDA for second year running
• *Nursing Times* Palliative Care Award
	• The extent of other independent contractors' systems development is unknown
	• Less known – not systematically collated at a PCT level – between primary and secondary care

ACTION	GROUP/PERSON RESPONSIBLE	DATE
• To further develop PALS – regular audit to monitor the effectiveness of the service	Head of Corporate Affairs	Ongoing✓
• To take part in the National Patient Surveys for PCTs and Mental Health	Head of Corporate Affairs	April/May 04✓
• To feed back results from the national surveys to staff and patients	Head of Corporate Affairs	June/July 04✓
○ Presentation at staff briefing		
○ Produce an article for *PCT World* (the PCT staff magazine, published on a monthly basis)	Head of Corporate Affairs	July 04✓
○ Place information on the PCT's shared folders (intranet)		
• To use the information gleaned from the national surveys to inform and influence how we deal with and involve patients and carers (action plan produced)	PPI Group	Dec 04✓
• To continue to use every opportunity to involve patient and carers	PPI Group	Ongoing✓
• To introduce a system to monitor pressure sore prevalence in the Community Hospitals	Head of Healthcare Governance	June 04✗
• To extend the regular patient satisfaction surveys in Primary Care and Community Hospitals	Head of Healthcare Governance	Sept 04✗
Work to create positive relationship with Primary Care Forum	PPI Group	Ongoing✓
• To further develop a cohesive PPI strategy for the PCT	Head of Corporate Affairs	Sept 04✓✓
• To increase staff awareness of PPI including independent contractors by holding workshops and training sessions	Head of Corporate Affairs	Sept 04✓
• To implement the new Complaints Procedure for patients	Complaints Manager	June 04✓
• To provide information and training on the new complaints procedure to staff including independent contractors	Complaints Manager	June 04✓
• To further develop closer links with the Community and Voluntary sectors particularly with 'hard to reach' groups	Head of Corporate Affairs	March 05

ACTION	GROUP/PERSON RESPONSIBLE	DATE
• To consider PPI on all PCT committees and groups (H & R Patient Forum members on RM & A & CG Sub-Committees)	Head of Corporate Affairs	June 04✓
• To actively seek patient involvement on each modernisation project	Head of Corporate Affairs	Ongoing✓
• To actively use information from complaints and PALS issues to learn as an organisation to improve the patient experience	Complaints Manager/Head of Corporate Affairs	Ongoing✓
• To engage with young people regarding their health issues and vulnerable (older and younger) people	Public Health Manager	Dec 04
• To share information about patient experience with local government organisations	Head of Corporate Affairs	Ongoing✓
• To further develop the links between PALS and Patient Forum	Head of Corporate Affairs	Ongoing✓
• Patient experience of commissioned services		

Section 2: Use of information

STRENGTHS	WEAKNESSES
• Strong performance management culture – much information on services commissioned from acute providers and Ambulance Trust	• Limited access to IT and clinical information for community clinicians
• Robust HR systems	• Little information on patient outcomes
• Good access to IT and the internet at headquarters	• Weak systems and mechanisms to feedback information to staff
• Robust IT infrastructure and rapidly developing data collection in Primary Care	• Information governance limited knowledge
• Regular clinical auditing undertaken in primary care and shared with the PCT	
• Regular complaints information to the Board	
• Caldicott Guardian in post	
• New IM&T team appointed	

ACTION	GROUP/PERSON RESPONSIBLE	DATE
• Improve methods of making information more accessible to staff		
○ Use of team briefing	Communications Manager	Ongoing✓ (Meet monthly)
○ Team meetings	Communications Manager and Head of Healthcare Governance	Quarterly✓ Sept 04✓
• Regular feature and articles in *PCT World*	Head of Healthcare Governance	
• Carry out an assessment of current information available	Communications Manager, Public Health Information Officer and Head of Healthcare Governance	
• Regular progress against implementation of the NHS IM&T Strategy	Head of IM&T	Quarterly✓ Sept 04✓
• Further refinement and development of a strategic approach to how we as a PCT use information	Communications Manager, Public Health Information Officer and Head of Healthcare Governance	
○ Establish a formal information group	and IM&T	Ongoing (group set up)✓
• Develop the concepts of Knowledge Management and Evidence Based Healthcare		
• Review IM&T development and strategy and disseminate widely	Head of IM&T	April 04✓
• Develop a Governance Section of the H & R PCT's website	Communications Manager and Head of Healthcare Governance	Sept 04✗
• Perform a baseline audit of Healthcare Records	Head of Healthcare Governance	March 04✓
• Provide training on Information Governance	Training and Education Manager	March 05

Section 3: Processes for quality improvement – risk management and incident reporting

STRENGTHS	WEAKNESSES
• Established Clinical Governance, Risk Management and Controls Assurance Sub-Committees • PCT has linked clinical and non-clinical governance via the concept of 'healthcare governance' • Small competent and skilled healthcare governance department established • Established 'Accident, Incident and Clinical Incident Reporting System', including near misses for all staff employed by the PCT • Community Pharmacy has piloted a drug error reporting system • Culture of significant incident reviewing development in primary care	• Variable incident reporting in primary care • Newly established immature organisation • Only limited reporting from independent contractors

ACTION	GROUP/PERSON RESPONSIBLE	DATE
• To further develop and strengthen health and safety arrangements and policies (HSE Visit)	Head of Healthcare Governance	Sept 04✔
• To continually monitor and implement relevant Controls Assurance action plans	Head of Healthcare Governance	Ongoing✔
• To review Accident, Incident and Clinical Incident Reporting Policy and gain PCT Board Approval	Head of Healthcare Governance	March 04✔
• To ensure that PCT is able to report all clinical incidents to the NPSA via the National Reporting and Learning System (NRLS)	Head of Healthcare Governance	Dec 04 (waiting for NPSA)

ACTION	GROUP/PERSON RESPONSIBLE	DATE
• To further develop the methods for feeding back summary information from the incident reporting system to managers and clinicians, including near misses	Head of Healthcare Governance	Ongoing✓
• To further develop risk management training programmes for all levels of staff within the organisation	Head of Healthcare Governance and Educ, Trg and Dev Manager	Ongoing✓
• To ensure eight appropriate senior managers/clinicians undertake root cause analysis training provided by the NPSA	Head of Healthcare Governance	Jan 05✓
• To work with independent contractors to reduce clinical risks – offer/share PCT policies and procedures	Head of Healthcare Governance	March 05✓
• Continue to work with community pharmacists to improve the drug prescribing and dispensing errors	Pharmaceutical Advisor	Ongoing✓
• To raise awareness of clinical risk management and incident reporting	RM and CA SC and Head of Healthcare Governance	Ongoing✓
• To hold a Governance Seminar focused on risk management and learning the lessons from clinical incidents		Jan 05

Section 4: Processes for quality improvement – research and development

STRENGTHS	WEAKNESSES
• Have developed a Research Governance Implementation Plan • Several GPs with special interest in research • TARGET days encourage research-based approach through the inclusion of targeted sessions • PCT is a member of a local Research Management team • Head of Healthcare Governance is a member of a local Research Governance Scientific Committee	• Little experience of primary research

ACTION	GROUP/PERSON RESPONSIBLE	DATE
• To raise the awareness of R&D within the PCT – consider cost implications	CG SC	March 04✓
• Ensure good links to Acute Trust's R&D function	Head of Healthcare Governance	Oct 04✗
• To establish a PCT R&D Group	Head of Healthcare Governance	Sept 04✗
• To continually monitor and review the PCT's Research Governance Implementation Plan	Clinical Governance Sub-Committee	Quarterly✓
• To establish a database of all research activity within the PCT	Clinical Audit and Effectiveness Facilitator	June 04✓
• To report regularly to the Clinical Governance Sub-Committee on research	Head of Healthcare Governance and R&D Group	Quarterly✓

Section 5: Clinical audit and clinical effectiveness

STRENGTHS	WEAKNESSES

• Well-established culture of clinical audit in Mental Health
  o Annual clinical audit programme
  o Regular meeting of most disciplines
  o Robust suicide audit
• Good but limited history of countywide audit for GPs
• Part of the countywide audit group developing NSF-based audits for CHD, diabetes and older people/stroke
• Established collaborative CHD modernisation group, consisting of primary and secondary care staff focused on the CHD NSF
• Employed a Clinical Audit and Effectiveness Facilitator responsible for progressing Clinical Audit and Effectiveness within the PCT
	• Suboptimal development of activity/capacity
	• Protected time for development of audit programmes
	• Access to online resources in clinical setting
	• Limited capacity of clinical effectiveness and audit skills

ACTION	GROUP/PERSON RESPONSIBLE	DATE
• To develop a clinical audit programme based on the national imperatives, i.e. NICE guidelines, the NSF and the LDP	Commissioning Team, Mental Health, CHD Modernisation Group, Prescribing Team Community Directorate	Ongoing✓
• Increase awareness and understanding of clinical audit by training and education	Head of Healthcare	March 04✓
○ Provide training to departments and directorates	Governance, CGSC and ED & T Group	Ongoing✓
○ Develop training strategy with EDT group and Library service	Clinical Audit and Effectiveness Facilitator (CA & CE) ED & T Group and Library Service	Ongoing✓
• Aim to get two clinical audit projects from each clinical area per year	CA and EF	Ongoing✓
• Include input from Expert Patient Programme	CA and EF/PPI Group	Oct 04✗
• Establishment of Clinical Audit database	CA and EF	March 04✓
• To ensure the involvement of patients and patient groups in establishing priorities for audit work at all levels and all parts of the process	CA and EF	Ongoing✓
• To produce a clinical audit and clinical effectiveness strategy for the PCT to be approved by the Clinical Governance Committee	CA and EF	April 04✓
• To produce an annual audit plan for the PCT	CA and EF	June 04✓
• To provide the clinical governance sub-committee with regular updates of progress with clinical audit	CA and EF	Ongoing✓
• To further encourage and facilitate clinical audit amongst independent contractors	CA and EF and ED & T Manager	Ongoing✓

ACTION	GROUP/PERSON RESPONSIBLE	DATE
• To link clinical audit in primary care with quality outcomes framework of the nGMS contract	CA and EF	Ongoing✓
• Establish a systematic approach to receiving, implementing and auditing NICE Guidelines	Head of Healthcare Governance, CA and EF Director of Public Health	Ongoing✓
• Continue to further develop an evidence-based culture	CA and EF	Ongoing
○ Clinical Effectiveness training day	CA and EF	Oct 04✓
• Baseline assessment of all primary care clinical areas, e.g. dentistry, physiotherapy, occupational therapy	Clinical Audit and Effectiveness Facilitator	Ongoing

Section 6: Complaints

STRENGTHS	WEAKNESSES
• Robust complaints system established with regular reports to the Board • Complaints manager in post • Robust policy • Meeting the NHS performance targets	• Not easy to link clinical incidents and other issues to complaints at present • Relationship – control of independent providers services e.g. NYED • No links to National Clinical Assessment Authority • Control of non-PCT staff – Out of Hours Service post 1 April 04

ACTION	GROUP/PERSON RESPONSIBLE	DATE
• To fully implement the new NHS Complaints Procedure	Complaints Manager	June 04✓
• To work in collaboration with other organisations to establish an integrated reporting and monitoring system	Incident reporting group and Head of Healthcare Governance	Ongoing✓
• To disseminate and share lessons leant from patient complaints throughout the PCT	Incident reporting group, Communications Manager	Ongoing✓
• To encourage and support primary care practitioners in the development of systems to manage complaints	Complaints Manager, Head of Primary Care, Head of Healthcare Governance	Ongoing✓
• To gather information regarding patient's experience of the complaints process in order to improve the system	Head of Corporate Affairs/ Complaints Manager	March 05
• To use the PCT prospectus to inform patients of system changes linked to complaints and the PCT's aim of local resolution nearest to the origin of the complaint	Head of Corporate Affairs/ Communications Manager	Dec 04✓
• To provide training on the new complaints procedure to a wide range of staff with emphasis on independent contractors	Complaints Manager	March 05
• To further develop links with partner organisations to aid the resolution of complex complaints	Complaints Manager	Ongoing✓

Section 7: Leadership, strategy and planning

STRENGTHS	WEAKNESSES
• Strong leadership from committed Board and managers • Introduced the concept of healthcare governance to converge clinical and non-clinical governance • Robust governance structure with clear lines of accountability • Non-executive directors chair the Clinical Governance and the Risk Management and Controls Assurance Sub-Committees • Director of Public Health and Head of Healthcare Governance are members of the local SHA clinical governance network • Strong communications policy • Communication manager in post	• The clinical governance structures and frameworks are still emerging

ACTION	GROUP/PERSON RESPONSIBLE	DATE
• Improved ownership from PEC and Board by participation in the NCGST Development Programme	PCT Board and Head of Healthcare Governance	Ongoing✓
• To build upon the learning from the National Clinical Governance Support Team (NCGST) and National Primary Care Trust Development Programme (Nat PACT) development programme		
• Continue to reinforce the visions and values of the PCT	Communications Manager	Ongoing✓
• To further develop links with PCTs in region	Head of Healthcare Governance	Aug 04✓

ACTION	GROUP/PERSON RESPONSIBLE	DATE
• To develop a clinical governance reporting template for clinical areas	Head of Healthcare Governance	Sept 04✗
• To raise awareness amongst the PCT staff and independent contractors by	Head of Healthcare Governance	Jan 04✓
○ Holding clinical governance seminars	Education and Training Group	Ongoing✓
○ Training and education to clinical areas		Ongoing✓
• Disseminate good practice – via publication and conferences	PPI group	Ongoing✓
• Further development of PALS	Head of Corporate Affairs	
• To conduct annual clinical governance visits to all GP practices – under the nGMS	Head of Healthcare Governance and Head of Primary Care	March 05
• To fully implement the recommendation of 'Assurance to the Board' and establish an integrated assurance framework	Director of Public Health, Director of Finance and Head of Healthcare Governance	March 05
• To ensure the PCT establishes a systematic approach to addressing the recommendations of the CHI and AC Review of the CHD NSF	Director of Public Health and Head of Healthcare Governance	May 04✓

Section 8: *Staff focus*

STRENGTHS	WEAKNESSES
• Open and honest culture • Robust and effective Joint Negotiating Committee (JNC) • JNC member on Trust Board • Staff appraisal scheme	• Communication remains challenging due to geographical spread of staff • Human resources training and development and organisational development strategies are being developed

STRENGTHS	WEAKNESSES
• Newly formed Education and Training committee • Regular staffing meeting • Team briefing • *PCT World* staff newsletter • High levels of staff involvement • IWL Pledge – Practice Award • Staff Handbook	• GP appraisal not fully bedded in – limited number of GP appraisers • New staff appraisal scheme not fully bedded in

ACTION	GROUP/PERSON RESPONSIBLE	DATE

• Review the results of annual staff survey – feed back to staff:
  o Team briefing
  o Clinical teams and localities
	Head of Healthcare Governance and Head of HR	April–June 04✓

• Production of staff charter	Head of HR	June/July 04✗
• Establishment of a communication group to set, monitor and improve communication within and without the organisation	Communications Manager	June/July 04✓
• Establish a system to monitor CPD and link to PDP – linked to a corporate development strategy for CPD and PDP	Head of HR	March 04✓
• To develop/establish a development programme for middle managers	Head of HR and Educ, Trg and Dev Manager	March 05✓
• To further develop and expand HR services to address the needs of GP practices as/if required	Head of HR	June 04✓
• To further develop and refine the role of the Education, Training and Development Group	Educ, Trg and Dev Manager	July 04✓
• Perform a training needs analysis	Head of HR and Educ, Trg and Dev Manager	March 05

Section 9: Commissioning of patient/care/services

STRENGTHS	WEAKNESSES
• Robust performance management system for access to secondary/tertiary services • Developing good working relationships with local Hospital NHS Trust (main secondary care provider) • Good access data from primary care (GP) • Good access CMD • Head of Healthcare Governance member of Acute and Ambulance Trusts Clinical Governance Committees • Regular reports on Commissioning Services presented at Public Trust Board every 2 months by Director of Strategy and Commissioning	• Little information on the quality and outcome of care provided by service commissioned • Limited robust information of the quality and outcome of care provided in the community by GPs and GDPs

ACTION	GROUP/PERSON RESPONSIBLE	DATE
• To ascertain the clinical governance arrangements of secondary and tertiary care providers	Head of Healthcare Governance	June 04✓
• To continue to develop quality indicators/outcomes. Output measure for our main secondary care providers (linked to the LDP)	Head of Healthcare Governance and IM&T Manager	Ongoing✓
• Establish formal clinical governance/framework meeting/arrangement with main secondary care providers and relevant Acute Trusts	Director of Public Health and Head of Healthcare Governance	Ongoing✓

• In collaboration with other PCTs to agree a joint approach to understanding the clinical governance arrangements of major healthcare providers	Head of Healthcare Governance	Ongoing✓
• To agree a joint approach with other PCTs with regard to clinical governance performance of major healthcare providers	Head of Healthcare Governance	Ongoing✓
• To establish mechanisms to agree priority area of mutual benefit to the PCT and provider organisations	Head of Healthcare Governance	Ongoing✓

Staff designations

Clinical Audit and Effectiveness Facilitator
Clinical Nurse Advisor, Mental Health Acute Services
Communications Manager
Complaints Manager
Director of Community Services
Education, Training and Development Manager
Head of Community Dental Services
Head of Corporate Affairs
Head of Healthcare Governance
Head of Human Resources
Head of Podiatry
Head of Primary Care
Information Management and Technology Manager
Mental Health General Manager
Pharmaceutical Advisor
PPI Group – Patient and Public Involvement Group
Professional Head of Clinical Psychology
Public Health Information Officer

Reference Department of Health: *The New NHS: Modern, Dependable.*

Appendix 4.2
An example of a personal development plan

CONFIDENTIAL

HOSPITAL . . . .

DIRECTORATE . . . .

Name:

Position:

PERSONAL AND PROFESSIONAL DEVELOPMENT PLAN

Date: From . . . .   To . . . .

Preceptor/supervisor . . . .

In order to achieve the compliance expected/required of a healthcare professional undertaking the role of venous cannulation within this organisation, the line manager (name) . . . . and staff member (name) . . . . performed a SWOT analysis of his current position on Date . . . . Time . . . .

Strengths	Weaknesses
• Confident • Competent • Time management • Enthusiastic • Committed • Adaptable to change • Relevant experience in taking charge of the ward	• Inexperience with cannulation • Had no formal education or training with regards to venous cannulation (see one do one)
Opportunity	**Threats**
• Access to personal development plan • Support and commitment to develop the role of venous cannulation • Support	• Clinical time versus personal time • Lack of time to attend courses on cannulation • Time on the ward • Perception of colleagues in light of the incident

Following the SWOT analysis, a personal and professional development programme was agreed. The agreement is as follows:

• to hold monthly reviews
• to document after each session with regards to progress (see monthly review sheet)

- any new training/development requirements will be identified and added and dated as identified.

HOSPITAL . . . .

DIRECTORATE

WARD

Personal and professional development programme for

NAME . . . .   **POSITION** . . . .

The following development plan has been discussed and agreed by

Name: . . . .   **Date:** . . . .   **Signature:** . . . .   **Date:** . . . .
Preceptor

Name: . . . .   **Date:** . . . .   **Signature:** . . . .   **Date:** . . . .
Preceptee

Identified training and development needs to be met by agreed competencies	Training and development method	Time-scale	Evaluation of training
To develop knowledge, understanding and skills associated with venous cannulation	To attend the in-house educating and training programme for venous cannulation To shadow a senior experienced clinician during cannulation To practise cannulation under supervision of an accredited trainer To participate in cannulation audit within the clinical area		

Hospital . . . .

Directorate . . . .

Ward . . . .

Personal and professional development plan for NAME . . . .

Monthly review

Date	Progress	Signature

Chapter 5

Identifying and Exploring the Barriers to the Implementation of Clinical Governance

Rob McSherry and Paddy Pearce

Introduction

Chapter 4 offered practical examples on how the clinical governance framework can be applied to an organisation, team and individual in the pursuit of clinical excellence. For some healthcare organisations, teams and professionals the issues affecting the implementation of clinical governance are not associated with what it is and how the key components relate to practice, but in resolving barriers associated with the demands of a busy daily practice, the balance between improving quality and achieving increasingly difficult and forever changing targets, financial difficulties and a real and perceived lack of organisational support in developing staff. This chapter explores the potential barriers affecting the implementation of clinical governance and how they can be resolved by focusing on models of change, teamwork, collaboration, partnerships, leadership and cultural issues.

The potential barriers affecting the implementation of clinical governance

Barriers are defined as 'an obstruction, a fence or wall, anything that holds apart or separates' (Collins 1987, p. 67).

Activity 5.1: Establishing the barriers to implementing clinical governance

Reflect upon Collins' (1987) definition of barriers and make a few notes regarding what you think the potential barriers are to implementing clinical governance in your area of work.

Compare your notes with the themes in the Feedback box at the end of the chapter.

It would appear that Collins' (1987) definition of barriers is out of context when exploring the barriers to clinical governance within healthcare organisations. The definition appertains to a physical presence which restricts movement. A critical review of this definition, however, shows quite the opposite.

Firstly, the word 'obstruction' refers to a blockage or anything that withholds or hinders the flow of something. If this term were linked to clinical governance, an obstruction would relate to anything that affects the quality of the vast array of systems and processes akin to its structures; for example, an obstruction in the channels of communication and information-giving between healthcare professionals and patients about pre-operative risks and benefits associated with a certain procedure; or the failure to document an incident in the patient's healthcare records after a fall, where the patient/family complain about the incident, asking for a full explanation several weeks after the event and no one can remember the event.

Secondly, a 'fence or wall' relates to boundaries, a term used frequently when exploring the relevance of clinical governance to healthcare organisations. Boundaries can be used as a means of protection or a barrier to be climbed. Within the context of clinical governance, boundaries should be used to safeguard the quality of the services.

Thirdly, 'holds apart or separates' suggests the need for dividing or keeping something apart for a specific purpose, whether this be for positive or negative reasons. Similarities emerge when relating this to clinical governance and the associated key components that are separate by name but not function; for example, the need for clinical risks to be detected so that clinical quality is improved or maintained.

It is evident from Collins' (1987) definition that barriers can be positive and negative in nature, which is of immense importance when exploring these issues within a healthcare organisation and the context of clinical governance. For example, the clinical governance framework could be viewed positively at organisational level because it provides a means to improve quality by developing its systems and processes, but for an individual in daily practice it may be viewed negatively because it is just another change without perceived relevance to his or her daily practices.

'It is important in the implementation process within a Trust (or other related healthcare organisations) that the requirements for and the process of clinical governance be viewed with enthusiasm rather than scepticism. It can really only be satisfactorily implemented on the basis of a welcomed initiative with the potential for developing real improvements in quality of patient care rather than a political imposition.' (Edwards & Packham 1999, p. 13)

For some healthcare organisations, teams and individuals this is not the perceived norm. Clinical governance is yet another 'thing' imposed by government in response to the poor media view of the NHS because of the high profile cases that have highlighted inadequate standards and practices – cases like the following:

- The Neale Enquiry (2004) – relating to a consultant gynaecologist who was found negligent for numerous surgical interventions resulting in unnecessary pain and suffering for his patients and their families (DH 2004a).
- The Bristol Case – a consultant paediatric surgeon was found to have death rates for paediatric heart surgery significantly higher than the national average, and this only became known as a result of whistle-blowing (*The Lancet* 1998).
- Alder Hey Children's Hospital – a consultant pathologist at the Royal Liverpool Children's Hospital, Alder Hey, Liverpool, removed the organs of over 2000 children without the consent of their parents. As a result of an inquiry he was banned from practising in the UK, and all NHS Acute Trusts had to perform a census of their pathology department and list retained organs. The Chief Medical Officer issued guidance on post-mortem examination (DH 2001a).
- The Shipman Enquiry (2001) – a general practitioner was convicted of the murder of 15 patients as a result of morphine poisoning (Ramsey 2001).
- The Alitt Enquiry – a qualified enrolled nurse working in a paediatric unit was convicted of murdering four children and injuring nine others (MacDonald 1996).

These are all cases that have affected the public's confidence in the UK NHS, a confidence that requires rebuilding. Put bluntly, clinical governance 'is much more than a set of bureaucratic systems' (Harvey 1998, p. 8); it is a framework which is designed to help doctors, nurses, therapists and indeed all healthcare staff to improve organisational, team and individual standards and quality of care. To achieve the aims of clinical governance – reducing clinical risks, promoting continuous quality improvement and providing the best practices based on the best evidence delivered by professionals who have the correct knowledge, skills and competence via a system of lifelong learning – a shift in attitudes and culture is needed to a positive view of clinical governance rather than a negative one. Cullen *et al.* (2000) states that we need to change the culture of healthcare organisation and to do this 'we need to unlearn some old habits and develop some new habits'. This view is supported by Davies *et al.* (2000) who states that we will need to 'change the way things are done around here 'to unlock the true potential of clinical governance'.

Box 5.1   The perceived barriers to implementing clinical governance

- Lack of understanding
- Fear
- No clear vision
- It's nothing new
- It's a passing fad
- Lack of time
- Lack of resources
- Tool of the management
- Lack of support
- Poor information/no information
- Poor leadership
- Ineffective communication

Note: This not an exhaustive list of the potential or perceived barriers to implementing clinical governance.

The barriers affecting the implementing process of clinical governance are vast but not insurmountable, as outlined in Box 5.1.

Box 5.1 shows that the barriers to implementing clinical governance originate from internal and external sources which can affect the organisation, teams and individuals, as illustrated in Fig. 5.1. These can be themed into several key areas, as outlined in Fig. 5.2 and discussed here.

Internal	External
Individual	**Individual**
• Lack of knowledge	• Lack of support, i.e. peer, management or organisational
• Lack of understanding	• Lack of resources, i.e. personnel
• Lack of confidence	• Lack of time
• Lack of ownership	• Ineffective communication
• Fear of what's about to be or is being left behind	• Information
• Resistance to change	
• Ineffective communication	
• Information	
Organisation	**Organisation**
• Culture: openness, trust	• Political pressure
• Leadership styles	• Increased demand on already overstretched services
• Lack of ownership	• Increased performance targets
• Management styles:	• Public expectations
– proactive/reactive	• Increased litigation
– change management	• Lack of resourcing, i.e. financial backing
• Ineffective communication	
• Information	

Fig. 5.1   Internal and external factors influencing the implementation of clinical governance.

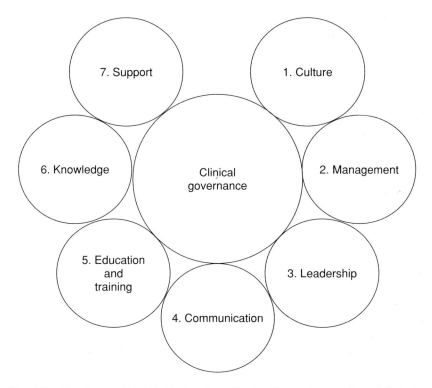

Fig. 5.2 Key themes linked to the barriers affecting the implementation of clinical governance.

Culture

What do we mean by culture? Culture is defined as 'the skills and arts, etc. of a given people in a given period; civilisation . . . improvements of the mind, manners, etc. . . . . development by special training or care' (Collins 1987, p. 214).

During the late 1990s and early 2000s the word culture has become more prominent within the NHS, perhaps as a result of the many failures of healthcare systems, processes and the high profile professional misconduct cases, as previously mentioned. A common theme that has emerged following the inquiries of the recent clinical disasters and CHI investigations (North Lakeland Healthcare NHS Trust) is the use of the word 'culture' or phrases like 'open or closed culture'. The questions posed by some healthcare professionals are:

- Why is creating the right culture important to the NHS?
- How do you go about creating the right culture for an organisation, team or individuals?

Table 5.1   Cultural barriers affecting the implementation of clinical governance.

Barriers	Rationale
● *Lack of openness*	● To encourage reporting of untoward incidents or practices. To state how you feel regarding a situation, whether it is good or not so good
● *Mistrust between employees and employers*	● To foster an environment where staff feel safe to whistle blow or voice concerns without retribution
● *Undervaluing staff*	● To create a feeling of confidence and pride in one's daily role and how that role relates to others, etc.
● *Not rewarding staff*	● Leads to low morale and inhibits the continuous quality improvements
● *Stifling innovation*	● Without nurturing continuous development the organisation and quality of care may not be developed and could deteriorate
● *Lack of transparency*	● Encouraging an openness where opinions within and external to the organisation are listened to

The Department of Trade and Industry (DTI 1997) suggests that an effective organisation recognises that shared culture, shared learning, shared effort and shared information are the keys to high productivity and quality. For clinical governance to become a reality for any healthcare organisation, the cultural barriers outlined in Table 5.1 need addressing, as the rationale column suggests.

A healthcare organisation that is innovative, involving staff from all levels of the organisation and patients/carers, is an ideal foundation for the implementation of clinical governance – an approach advocated by Haslock (1999):

'for clinical governance to raise standards in a genuine and lasting fashion it must be developed in a supportive, blame-minimising, educational atmosphere'.

Table 5.2 Types of culture (adapted from Hawkins and Shohet (1989) in Northcott (1999)).

Type	Key attribute	Preferred culture in achieving the modernisation of the NHS via clinical governance (the more asterisks the higher the preference)
Blame	A culture that seeks to address mistakes and apportions blame to individuals	*
Bureaucratic	An over-reliance on rules, regulations, procedures and policies at the jeopardy of individual personal judgement	* *
Mistrust (watch your back)	An over-competitive environment that seeks to embarrass departments and individuals and stifles developments	*
Reactive (knee-jerk)	Short-term management plans and dealing with the immediate problem. No long-term vision	*
Proactive (learning)	Encouraging learning and development. Learning from mistakes.	* * * * *

The challenge for some healthcare organisations, teams and individuals is how to develop this culture within their respective workplace. The starting point for addressing the questions associated with culture is to establish the type of culture within your present organisation or team. Hawkins and Shohet (1989) identify five types of culture, as outlined in Table 5.2.

It is clear from Table 5.2 that a transformational culture is 'a construct that describes the nature of an effective culture' (Manley 2005, p. 62). In order for healthcare governance to occur, a proactive transformational culture of learning is the most suitable for the implementation of a system of clinical governance. This is because an environment or culture that seeks to apportion blame only leads to secrecy, mistrust and a failure to report mistakes, with a knee-jerk reaction to resolving the incidents; for example, a healthcare professional administers the wrong medication to a patient, which results in no harm to the patient. The immediate response of management was to discipline the member of staff, who received a written warning on his/her personal file – a classic case of reactive knee-jerk culture that actively seeks to apportion blame because of failure to adhere rigidly to policy and procedure. This example demonstrates the element of culture that is bureaucratic, reactionary and closed, by blaming individuals.

Alternatively, in an open learning or proactive culture the incident would have been dealt with by exploring and establishing the facts before apportioning blame, with the systems and processes reviewed before any action was taken against the individual. This approach treats the whole incident as a learning opportunity for the individual and the organisation and where possible offers support, if needed, to the individual and patient concerned. The lessons learned from the incident are disseminated throughout the organisation, in an anonymous way to avoid naming, blaming and shaming of individuals, to avoid recurrence of this type of event. The National Patient Safety Agency (NPSA) publication 'The Manchester Patient Safety Framework (MaPSaF)' (NPSA 2006) offers a typology of safety cultures, as shown in Table 5.3, which complement the works of Hawkins and Shohet (1989). The framework by Parker and Hudson (2001) builds upon the work of Westrum (1992).

It is evident from Tables 5.2 and 5.3 that for healthcare governance to succeed, an environment is necessary that is open, honest, trusting and willing to learn from its mistakes and share good practices. The preferred culture to promote this type of environment is that of a 'transformation and constructive culture', a culture that:

- Promotes learning
- Learns from experiences and mistakes
- Communicates to all
- Collaborates between all levels of the organisation
- Rewards, values and develops staff at all levels
- Is genuinely committed to the continuous improvement of patient services
- Values diversity and treats all as equal partners

This type of open or transparent culture takes 'time, and requires working for collaborative results rather than relying upon domination or

Table 5.3 The Manchester Patient Safety Framework (MaPSaF). Reprinted with kind permission from the University of Manchester (2006).

A	**Pathological:** organisation with a prevailing attitude of 'why waste our time on safety' and, as such, there is little or no investment in improving safety
B	**Reactive:** organisations that are serious about patient safety after an incident has occurred
C	**Bureaucratic:** organisations that are very paper-based and safety involves ticking boxes to prove to auditors and assessors that they are focused on safety
D	**Proactive:** organisations that place a high value on improving safety, actively invest in continuous safety improvements and reward staff who raise safety-related issues
E	**Generative:** the nirvana of all safety organisations in which safety is an integral part of everything that they do. In a generative organisation, safety is truly in the hearts and minds of everyone, from senior managers to front line staff

compromise as a quick fix' (Northcott 1999, p. 10). Some organisations will require a cultural change to successfully implement clinical governance. This will not be easy and will require careful management and good leadership.

Management

The management style of a healthcare organisation will have a significant impact on how clinical governance is perceived and implemented. Management and leadership go hand in hand, but there is a difference between the two. Marquis and Hutson (2000) suggest that management is about guiding and directing staff and resources and is concerned with having the power and legitimate authority for particular tasks and duties. Essentially management is primarily concerned with outcomes and the manipulation of resources to achieve the desired outcome(s). For example, in relation to clinical governance the chief executives of healthcare organisations are accountable to parliament for the implementation of the clinical governance framework, ensuring clinical quality along with meeting financial and performance targets – targets such as those outlined in the Standards for Better Health (DH 2004b) and the Annual Health Check (Healthcare Commission 2005), and those existing targets such as patients being seen in the Accident and Emergency department within four hours of arrival or being seen by a consultant within 13 weeks from the time of GP referral. These are all standards that require achievement through the process of delegation to other personnel within the organisation.

Management in this instance is about the transferring of roles and responsibilities to a specified team or individual in order to achieve the specific standards or desired aims and objectives. This collaborative and participative approach to management is the type that encourages a shared responsibility and ownership of what the organisation is trying to achieve. This is an essential attribute in the development, implementation and monitoring of clinical governance, where the success of the systems and processes as outlined in Chapters 3 and 4 is strongly associated with the specific management style of the lead for that part of the service. For example, if the manager or lead clinician is autocratic and not prepared to listen to the opinions of others, this will have a detrimental effect on advancing the quality improvement programme.

Previously in the NHS, effective management was valued more than good leadership. 'In difficult times, people need leadership as well as management' (Stewart 1996, p. 3) – an approach advocated within the NHS of today in addressing the factors that have led to the introduction of clinical governance and in developing new and creative ways of implementing the key systems and processes akin to clinical governance. In this instance management is crucial in both highlighting key leaders to take on the roles and responsibilities for advancing clinical governance and in empowering them to do this effectively without managerial interference. The National Clinical Governance Support Team (NCGST) (http://www.cgsupport.nhs.uk/) provides a variety of clinical governance development programmes for team and NHS staff to attend (NCGST). So what is the preferred management style for achieving clinical governance?

Management styles and clinical governance

Several theories have influenced the management of the NHS (Marquis & Hutson 2000). These can be categorised into three broad headings that have some degree of applicability to the implementation of clinical governance because of the nature of the management style used; see Table 5.4, adapted from Marquis and Hutson (2000).

It is evident from Table 5.4 that for clinical governance to be successfully implemented a combination of the three main management styles

Table 5.4   Management styles and their applicability to clinical governance.

Theory	Description	Applicability to clinical governance
Scientific management	• Based on scientific principles • Efficient and effective use of resources • Having the appropriate staff and qualifications • Retaining and developing the staff • Valuing and rewarding staff • Cooperative relationships between managers and personnel	This management style is suited to the development of clinical governance because it links nicely to the notion of performance management. Performance management is associated with the continuous development and rewarding of staff.
Management functions	• Planning • Commanding • Controlling • Coordinating • Organising • Staffing • Directing • Reporting	This type of management style is essentially related to the core aspects of the clinical governance framework because it fits in with almost all of the key components. For example, command and control are associated with 'accountability'. Staffing and reporting are associated with performance management and clinical risk. The planning and coordinating are related to quality improvement.
Human relationships management	• Involving staff • Valuing staff • Staff participation • Involved and shared decision-making	This management style pertains to the humanistic element of clinical governance and the notion of working in teams, sharing and learning from each when things go well or not so well, along with the involvement of the patients who are viewed as an essential asset when developing clinical governance.

needs to be applied at organisation and team levels. Each organisation or team should consider what its current management style is and what is the best way forward for it to manage clinical governance for the future.

The difficulty for some healthcare organisations and staff is not in eliciting what the preferred management style is or ought to be, but in overcoming the barriers associated with managing change effectively. For some healthcare professionals clinical governance is a challenging concept that is associated with the reviewing of existing and the development of new systems and processes requiring change at all levels of the organisation. To this end the success of clinical governance will depend on how this change is managed. The following sections on change management and reaction to change are based on McSherry and Simmons (2001), with kind permission of Routledge, an imprint of Taylor & Francis Publishing Group.

Change management

Change is a complex process in which barriers are inherent, threatening the successful implementation of clinical governance. Utilising a change model can help guide the change process and help to reduce obstacles which may be encountered. Lewin (cited in Allen 1993) proposes a change model, the 'Force Field Theory', that has three fundamental stages – unfreezing, moving, refreezing – which could be useful when exploring the potential effects of introducing clinical governance within an organisation or team or for an individual.

Unfreezing. For change to occur, individuals need to recognise that there is a need for change. Lewin suggests that for unfreezing to occur there is a need to understand the driving and restraining forces that exist. For example, a driving force may be the limited availability of information to support a change in practice and the restraining forces could be negative attitudes from the staff about this aspect of not informing them what is going on. This is a potentially huge barrier to clinical governance, where staff are expected to operate within the systems and processes but have not been informed about them or what their roles and responsibilities are within them. Whilst these forces remain in balance the situation will remain in the status quo. Unfreezing of a situation can occur when driving forces are increased and restraining forces decreased.

Moving. This is where the organisation, team or individual begins to explore and examine the change or begins to accept or adjust to the changes being implemented. Teamwork needs to be nurtured and the emergence of key roles and responsibilities within the team highlighted.

For clinical governance to work effectively staff need to be informed, and involved with the change processes. Management therefore has a duty and responsibility in ensuring these actions occur.

Refreezing. Refreezing often occurs after a time, when the change has been accepted within the organisation or team and the individual staff settle back into a functional unit, where key roles and responsibilities are adopted, supported and communicated to and from each other.

Having decided upon the model of change to be used, it is essential to be aware of how individuals may react or respond to the plans to implement the clinical governance frameworks.

Reaction to change

Most healthcare professionals find change disruptive and by merely exposing the flaws of a particular practice or presenting research findings to support the rationale for change, you will still most likely face resistance. While individuals may resist, different people will respond differently. There are four main reasons why people resist change, as shown in Table 5.5.

The potential varied responses by individuals to a change are vast but should not be overlooked when implementing change on a scale as large as that required for the successful implementation of clinical governance. Managers should try to establish the views and opinions of the organisation, team and individuals about the levels of tolerance, misunderstanding and interest in clinical governance so that the barriers to change can be avoided. The combination of effective management with leadership may help this process, as will be explored in the next section.

Leadership

Many people confuse management and leadership. Before we can proceed we need to understand the differences and relationships between leadership and management. This was eloquently described by Field Marshall Slim:

> 'There is a difference between leadership and management. Leadership is of the spirit, compounded of personality and vision; its practice is an art. Management is of the mind, a matter of accurate calculation . . . its practice is a science. Managers are necessary; leaders are essential.'
> (Slim 1996, in Stewart 1996)

Table 5.5   Four main reasons for resisting change (adapted from Kotter and Schlesinger (1979) in McSherry *et al.* (2001)).

Type	Description
Parochial self interest	Where individuals may resist because they fear they may lose something they value as a result of the change.
Misunderstanding and lack of trust	Individuals often resist change because they do not understand its implications and perceive it might cost them more than they have to gain. This may occur where there is trust lacking between the person initiating the change and the workforce.
Different assessments	Individuals may assess the situation differently from those initiating the change and see more costs than benefits as a result, not only for themselves but for the organisation as a whole.
Low tolerance for change	Individuals may fear they will not be able to develop the new skills or behaviour needed after the change.

As mentioned in the previous section, managers are essential for the efficiency and effectiveness of an organisation and team. However, this is not to say that all good managers show the attributes that make successful leaders. For clinical governance to work we need leaders who can 'make others feel that what they are doing matters and hence make them feel good about their work (Stewart 1996, p. 4). Mullally (2001) advances Stewart's (1996) work about leaders by incorporating the need for a moral and ethical dimension to leadership. This notion of empowering, involving and valuing staff is fundamental in developing the culture in which clinical governance will operate effectively. The essential attributes of an effective clinical leader are that he/she is:

- A visionary
- A communicator
- A facilitator
- An advocator

- A critical thinker
- A doer
- An evaluator
- A motivator
- Respectable
- Knowledgeable
- Tactful
- Considerate
- Ethical
- Trustworthy
- Credible

A clinical leader will utilise these essential attributes to influence and develop the organisation, team and individuals by the execution of a specific leadership style, which can be summarised into four main types, as illustrated in Table 5.6.

Table 5.6 describes how a transformational and democratic leadership style is potentially the most suited to implementing a clinical governance framework. The issue for some organisations, teams and individuals is in establishing their leadership traits and how to address them. Table 5.7 offers examples of personality types (based on Allen (1993) and Lancaster and Lancaster's (1982) adaptation of Rogers and Shoemaker's example of personality types, used in McSherry and Simmons (2001)), with their traits and applicability to clinical governance.

Table 5.7 shows that the innovators would come out top for supporting the implementation of clinical governance. However, it is important to mention here that an organisation or team requires a combination and harmonisation of all of these personality types to achieve success. It would be impossible to develop a service if all involved were laggards or rejecters; likewise, if everyone were innovators who were never really challenged about their ideas or introductions of new systems and processes, this could result in advancing practices based on a minority opinion. To advance this work the NHS Leadership Qualities Framework (NHS Leadership Centre 2002) offers five personal qualities of leaders that are useful when introducing clinical governance. These are as follows:

(1) Self belief
(2) Self awareness
(3) Self management
(4) Drive for improvement
(5) Personal integrity

When considering introducing or changing systems and processes associated with healthcare governance it is important to consider personality

Table 5.6   Leadership style and applicability to clinical governance (adapted from Marquis and Hutson (2000)).

Theory	Description	Applicability to clinical governance
Authoritarian	• Strong control • Gives commands • Communicates downwards only • Does not involve others in decision-making • Apportions blame	This type of leadership is destructive and inappropriate for the implementation of clinical governance. The whole style is at variance with the openness and sharing of clinical governance philosophy.
Democratic	• Less control • Directs by guidance • Two way process of communication up and down • Shared decision-making • Uses constructive criticism	This is the preferred leadership style for implementing clinical governance. It offers a strong vehicle for breaking down the barriers by the development of a collaborative, empowering and trusting culture based on a bedrock of communication and partnership.
Laissez-faire	• Little control • Limited direction • Communicates well • Devolves decision-making • Group orientated • Does not criticise	This style, whilst containing some elements central to the development of a clinical governance culture, is not without its limitations. Constructive criticism is necessary with the clinical governance framework.

traits and qualities. The methods or changes advocated may or may not be the best way forward on this occasion. It is important to determine what is best for the team or individuals. The way forward in exploring the issues associated with implementing clinical governance is to seek the views and opinions of the staff. To ensure this occurs effectively, efficient channels of communication need to be operational.

Communication

As previously mentioned in Chapter 3, 'communication seems to be about an interaction where two or more people send and receive messages, and

Table 5.7 Personality types and traits (adapted from McSherry and Simmons (2001)).

Personality type	Personality traits	Applicability to clinical governance (the more asterisks, the more applicable)
Innovators	Curious, enthusiastic and eager.	* * * * *
Early adapters	Moderately enthusiastic, well-established group members, with high self-esteem. (Do not usually introduce radical/controversial ideas)	* * * *
Early majority	Accept the innovation just before the majorities do.	* * *
Late majority	View the innovation with scepticism, do not actively resist.	* *
Laggards	Suspicious of change, discourage others by their negative attitude.	*
Rejecters	Openly reject change and encourage others to do so.	*

in the process both present themselves and interpret the other' (McSherry 1999, p. 198). McSherry's quotation about communication relates to the need for a system of clinical governance because, 'without clear communication, it is impossible to give care effectively, make decisions with clients and families, protect clients from threats to well-being, coordinate and manage client care, assist the client in rehabilitation, offer comfort, or teach' (Potter & Perry 1993, p. 24). Effective communication is an integral ingredient for the success or failure of clinical governance. It is of paramount importance in ensuring effective communications between and within:

- The various systems and processes associated with the key components akin to clinical governance
- Individual healthcare professionals both clinical and non-clinical

- Organisations such as Primary Care Trusts, Strategic Health Authorities, Acute Trusts, the National Institute For Health and Clinical Excellence, Healthcare Commission, Department of Health
- Professional regulating bodies
- Non-statutory organisations
- Voluntary organisations.

A failure in communication between or within these organisations, teams or individuals could result in complaints about healthcare, which are in the main linked to a failure in communications associated with 'staff attitudes, poor inter-team communication or lack of information for patients' (O'Neill 2000, p. 817). For the systems and processes associated with clinical governance to work in harmony, it is vital to have a culture that encourages open channels of communication between and within all levels of the organisation, teams and individuals. Failures to actively encourage honesty, openness and 'freedom of speech' contradict the philosophy behind clinical governance of promoting an environment where clinical excellence will flourish. 'Whistle blowing' and the reporting of poor practices, performance or competencies associated with the systems, processes or individuals should be encouraged via open two-way channels of communication between all levels of the organisation.

Communication can be enhanced and improved in the clinical environment by:

- Sharing of goals
- Information
- Learning
- Roles and responsibilities.

In this way a culture based on teamwork, partnerships and mutual collaboration becomes the norm. Clinical governance is not designed to work in a unidisciplinary manner; it needs teams and the individuals within the teams to collaborate, reliant on the efficiency and effectiveness of the communication process.

Healthcare, and indeed clinical governance, is team-based, relying on the 'direct or indirect support and influences of others, either from their own or other professions or work groups' (Northcott 1999).

This point is highlighted by the NHS Circular 1999/065 where multidisciplinary and multiagency collaboration is viewed as an essential component for improving the efficiency and effectiveness of the health service. Effective team working and multidisciplinary or multiagency approaches to care delivery are only truly effective where communication is continuous and seamless. For example, it would be fair to state that a patient's recovery from stroke is interdependent on multidisciplinary collaboration and effective communications, not individual practices. For clinical governance to function efficiently and effectively healthcare professions need to have the ability to coordinate patient/carers' care by passing information to and fro within the multidisciplinary team, a skill which requires effective management and leadership qualities.

If we find it difficult to communicate effectively with each other and with patients, what can one expect to find when it comes to reviewing standards and when faced with the challenge of implementing clinical governance into organisation, team or individual practices? For clinical governance to succeed it becomes evident that communication is of paramount importance as it is the unifying factor that crosses through all the key components. Communications should be based on the following principles:

- Appreciation and understanding of individual roles and responsibilities.
- Open channels of communication between and within the organisation, teams and individuals.
- An ability to:
  - actively listen
  - express concerns
  - trust
  - work in teams
  - develop partnerships
  - collaborate
  - respond
  - act.

To achieve effective communications in supporting the implementation of the clinical governance framework the organisation, teams and individuals need to be adequately informed. The latter can only be achieved by offering the appropriate education and training.

Education and training

The education and training needs of healthcare professionals should be considered on a NHS-wide basis to inform and educate staff at all levels of the organisation about clinical governance. The education and training of all NHS personnel should be based on a 'need to know basis', where the appropriate information is provided about how clinical governance affects the individual and his or her role. To ensure that this happens, the employee and employer have a mutual responsibility to ensure that education and training are provided at a local level. Employees should make it known through their individual personal development plans what education and training they need to reflect the Agenda for Change (AfC) requirements (DH 2004c) and be linked to the Knowledge and Skills Framework (KSF) (DH 2004d) for their job profile. This process will ensure relevant training needs and competences are developed in a systematic and logical way commensurate with the clinical governance frameworks. The employer should seek to establish the educational needs of his or her employees, perhaps through the development and implementation of a staff 'clinical governance awareness questionnaire'. Likewise local universities providing healthcare courses need to develop clinical governance modules to educate both their pre- and post-registration healthcare students about clinical governance. The education and training programme(s) should be designed to best suit the target audience, as highlighted in Fig. 5.3.

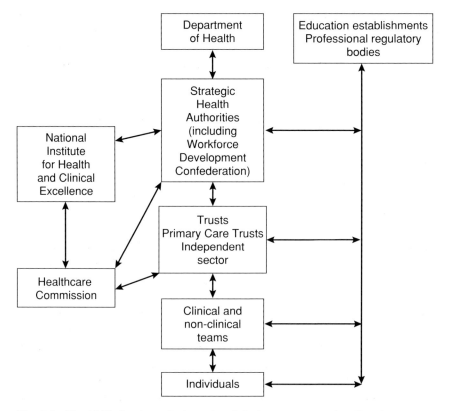

Fig. 5.3   The NHS structures that require clinical governance educational awareness sessions.

Figure 5.3 demonstrates the links between the various structures of the NHS and the need for education and training on clinical governance. It is imperative that all levels of the NHS are aware of their educational responsibilities in informing and educating their staff about the what and why of clinical governance and how it can make a difference to and for people.

The National Institute for Clinical Excellence (NICE) also has a responsibility to inform staff of the new guidelines to practice, in keeping with the philosophy of clinical governance. Similarly, the Commission for Health Improvements (CHI) and its successor organisation the Healthcare Commission have a responsibility for reviewing the effectiveness of clinical governance arrangements for all NHS Trusts and PCTs, in the course of which the provision and effectiveness of education and training will be assessed. The most difficult aspect in the education and training of clinical governance, we believe, is in linking it to the organisation, teams and individuals and in releasing personnel from their daily clinical duties to attend clinical governance education courses, etc. (Phipps 2000). For this to be effective the boards of the NHS organisations need to be committed and supportive with both monetary and other resources to enable and empower staff to embrace governance to be practised (Bevington *et al.* 2004).

Informing the organisation, team and individuals about clinical governance

The education and training needs of staff should be provided at three levels within a local healthcare organisation, where the information about clinical governance is designed with a specific targeted audience in mind. For example:

- At an organisational level all new employees of the Trust should attend the induction programme where a presentation on clinical governance should be given, associated with an overview of the structures and processes linked to clinical governance.
- At a team/directorate level a specific education and training programme could be delivered via the 'rolling development programmes' where clinical governance is aligned to the specific activities of the team. Case studies, critical reflections and reviews of complaints are used as examples of where clinical governance fits in with practice, accompanied by networking and sharing good and not so good practices within the teams and organisations and where necessary externally with other organisations.

- At an individual level the education and training needs of the individual should be associated with learning needs established after the performance review, forming the basis of the personal development plan linked to the AfC and KSF. This could be attendance on courses, seminars or workshops.

The barrier for some organisations, teams and individuals is in establishing what they need to know – i.e. where clinical governance relates to them and their practices – and in accessing the information on clinical governance. This is where having a knowledge and understanding of clinical governance is essential if it is to become an integral part of healthcare professions' daily practice and not seen to be another obstacle to practice.

Knowledge

To ensure that all healthcare staff have sufficient knowledge and understanding of clinical governance the education and training should be targeted to specific audiences with relevant aims and objectives that relate to and reflect the realities of their clinical or non-clinical practice. All NHS employees should be made aware of the idea that for clinical governance to become a reality, it is everybody's business. Clinical governance will only become a reality by engaging and using its frameworks. To make certain that clinical governance becomes known and owned by all NHS staff, educational and training programmes need to be directed to the appropriate audiences. The educational programmes on clinical governance need to cover the key components such as risk management, performance management, quality improvement, information and communication, accountability, patient and public involvement. Relevant examples and case studies are taken from real life situations to reinforce understanding and the relevance of clinical practice to employee's own practice.

The development of any educational programme for teams or individuals should be linked to demands of the local organisation or educational requirement highlighted via the Workforce Development Confederations, which are currently part of the Strategic Health Authorities. Any devised educational programmes should be:

- Multiprofessional
- Collaborative in nature
- Practically focused
- Evidence based
- Utilising a variety of teaching and learning methods

- Competency based
- Evaluated regularly
- Accredited by local universities, where possible.

An education programme could be based on the example in Box 5.2.

Box 5.2 Example education programme

Aim: to provide an introduction to clinical governance.

Learning outcomes:

- To describe what is meant by clinical governance
- To describe the key processes and components of clinical governance
- To describe what clinical governance means in relation to individual practice
- To apply the concept of clinical governance to clinical case studies identified from practice
- To locate evidence of and sources of information on clinical governance
- To evaluate the effectiveness of the course on the individual's understanding of clinical governance in relation to his or her practice.

All clinical governance educational programmes should be about learning from the practical experience gained in the workplace, with the learning shared and disseminated across multiprofessional boundaries. This approach to shared and problem-based learning is more likely to be successful, an approach advocated by the following statements:

> 'Learning in teams, developing multidisciplinary education and training across different agencies, is the way forward for creating learning environments. It will encourage healthcare professionals to work in partnerships in sharing ideas and solving problems that focus on what is important for patients.' (Squire 2000, p. 1015)

> 'New approaches to undergraduate medical education, such as the introduction of problem based learning, joint education with other professional disciplines, should in time improve teamworking skills; the importance of team working has been emphasised by the General Medical Council.' (Scally & Donaldson 1998, p. 65)

To foster this approach to shared learning and problem solving relating to the development, implementation, monitoring and evaluation of clinical governance, healthcare organisations, teams and individuals need to be supported.

Internal	External
Financial	**Locally**
• Funding for staff support and equipment, e.g. clinical audit, personnel etc.	• Collaboration with other healthcare agencies and patient/carers support groups
• Back fill costs for staff attending courses	• Developing partnerships with universities, education establishments
• The development of courses	
Resources	**Nationally**
• Education	• Links to the:
• Supervision	– Department of Health
• Time out	– Healthcare Commission
• Access to information	– NICE
• Expert and practical advice	– Professional regulatory bodies
• Accommodation	– National Patient Safety Agency
• Equipment	– Clinical Governance Support Team
• Support from management	
• Trust board commitment	

Fig. 5.4 Internal and external factors supporting clinical governance.

Support

The success of clinical governance will depend on the support and resources given within the various levels of the NHS to implement such a wide-ranging system. We believe that the support falls into two categories, internal and external, as highlighted in Fig. 5.4.

Figure 5.4 shows how the supporting infrastructures for the successful implementation of clinical governance depend on collaboration, partnerships and adequate levels of resourcing at organisational, team and individual level and effective communication. The support is not just about financial backing but the physical releasing of staff to develop their knowledge, understanding, skills and competence to deliver the clinical governance agenda at a local or individual level. Local support for staff could be in the form of:

- *Clinical supervision*: offering a framework for staff to identify and explore issues about the quality of care delivered, along with the identification of education and training needs in enabling them to improve their clinical competence.
- *Reflective practice and critical incident analysis*: to help identify and resolve clinical concerns and share good practice.

- *Lifelong learning*: the need to ensure that staff have the support to continuously develop professionally.
- *Performance management review*: to offer support and advice in the organisation's drive for continuous quality improvement.
- *Clinical audit*: to support staff in the evaluation of care associated with set standards and guidelines.
- *Offering the opportunity for networking and collaboration*: to encourage staff to share and learn from each other.
- *Professional self-regulation*: offering support and encouragement for development of the performances of the professions and individuals as outlined by the National Clinical Assessment Authority.

National support comes in the form of:

- *The National Institute for Clinical Excellence*: by setting clear national standards to provide clear guidance to the NHS on clinical and cost effectiveness across a wide range of health interventions, and the development of services.
- *National service frameworks*: directed at raising national standards of care and reducing unacceptable variations in care provision, e.g. coronary heart disease, mental health.
- *The Healthcare Commission*: to provide support by independently reviewing local efforts to improve the quality of healthcare by the implementation of the clinical governance systems and processes (DH 2001b).
- *The National Patient Safety Agency*: designed to support and develop learning from patient safety incidents.
- *The National Health Service Litigation Authority*: provides information and standards (CNST) on risk management, legal advice and claims handling.
- *The National Institute for Mental Health*: provides advice, guidance and best available evidence for mental health practice.
- *National Clinical Governance Support Team*: provides expert advice and a series of development programmes for NHS boards and clinical teams.

Without the correct and adequate local and national support for staff, to assist with their endeavours at an organisation, team and individual level to introduce clinical governance, the implementation and evaluation of clinical governance will not happen. Perhaps this accounts for the government's section in the National Plan in 2000 which states the 'NHS will support and value its staff' (DH 2000, p. 4), directed towards resolving the fundamental barriers associated with the provision of support.

Activity 5.1: Feedback: Establishing the barriers to implementing clinical governance

The barriers associated with the implementation of clinical governance can be classified into seven themes:

- Culture
- Management
- Leadership
- Communication
- Education and training
- Knowledge
- Support

By exploring these barriers, which tend to be viewed negatively, it is possible to develop positive strategies for the successful implementation of clinical governance systems and processes at an organisation, team and individual level.

Conclusion

This chapter shows how the implementation of clinical governance depends on resolving the potential barriers that exist within the organisation, teams and individuals – barriers that, if left unresolved, will make the linking of the systems and processes associated with the implementation of clinical governance difficult to achieve. These barriers can be classified into key themes associated with culture, management, leadership, communication, education and training, knowledge and support. As individual healthcare professionals, it is imperative that we understand the existence of these barriers and develop strategies to overcome them. Failure to embrace this challenge will make clinical governance difficult to implement in our daily practices.

Key points

The barriers to clinical governance:

- Refer to an obstruction or blockage in one or several of the complex systems and processes that make up clinical governance
- Can be classified as internal and external factors attributed to individuals or organisations

- Can be themed into seven key headings, strategies for which require development in resolving their impact at an organisation, team and individual level: culture, management, leadership, communication, education and training, knowledge, and support.

- Management, leadership styles and culture are three barriers which cannot be overlooked at either an organisation, team or individual level when considering the implementation of clinical governance.
- A closer inspection of these barriers will offer positive and constructive ways of achieving clinical governance.

- Adequate support is necessary.
- Education and training for staff on clinical governance are essential.

Suggested reading

Department of Health (2001) Assuring the Quality of Medical Practice: Implementing Supporting Doctors Protecting Patients. DH, London.
Stewart, R. (1996) Leading in the NHS: A Practical Guide, 2nd edn. Macmillan Business, London.

References

Allen, A. (1993) Changing Theory in Nursing Practice. *Senior Nurse*, 13 (1) 43–44.
Bevintong, J., Halligan, A. & Cullun, R. (2004) Understanding organisations: part 2. *Hospital Doctor*, 8 July.
Collins, W. (1987) *Collins Universal English Dictionary*. Readers Union Ltd, Glasgow.
Cullen, R., Nichols, S. & Halligan, A. (2000) NHS support team. Reviewing a service – discovering the unwritten rules. *British Journal of Clinical Governance*, 5 (4) 233–239.
Davies, H.T.O., Nutley, S.M. & Mannion, R. (2000) Organizational culture and quality of health care. *Quality in Health Care*, 9, 111–119.
Department of Health (2000) *National Plan*. DH, London.
Department of Health (2001a) *Interim Guidance on Post-Mortem Examination*. http://www.dh.gov.uk/PublicationsAndStatistics/LettersAndCirculars/DearColleagueLetters/DearColleagueLettersArticle/fs/en?CONTENT_ID=4002881&chk=ZJnu8d.
Department of Health (2001b) *Assuring the Quality of Medical Practice: Implementing Supporting Doctors Protecting Patients*. DH, London.

Department of Health (2004a) *Committee of Inquiry to Investigate How the NHS Handled Allegations About the Performance and Conduct of Richard Neale.* DH, London.

Department of Health (2004b) *Standards for Better Health: Healthcare Standards for Services Under the NHS – A Consultation Document.* DH, London.

Department of Health (2004c) *Agenda for Change – What Will it Mean for You? A Guide for Staff.* DH, London.

Department of Health (2004d) *The Knowledge and Skills Framework (NHSKSF) and Development Review Process (October 2004).* DH, London.

Department of Trade and Industry (1997) *Partnership with People.* DTI, London.

Edwards, J. & Packham, R. (1999) A model for the practical implementation of clinical governance. *Journal of Clinical Excellence*, 1 (1) 13–18.

Harvey, G. (1998) Improving patient care. *RCN Magazine*, Autumn, 8–9.

Haslock, I. (1999) Introducing clinical governance in an acute trust. *Hospital Medicine*, 60 (10) 745–747.

Hawkins, S. & Shohet, R. (1989) *Supervision in the Helping Professions.* Open University Press, Milton Keynes.

Healthcare Commission (2005) *Annual Health Check.* http://www. healthcarecommission.org.uk/serviceproviderinformation/annualhealthcheck.cfm.

Jasper, M. & Jumma, M. (2005) *Effective Healthcare Leadership.* Blackwell Publishing, Oxford.

Lancaster, J. & Lancaster, W. (1982) *The Nurse as the Change Agent.* Mosby, St Louis.

The Lancet (1998) Editorial. First lessons from the 'Bristol case'. *The Lancet*, 351, 117, 1669.

MacDonald, A. (1996) Responding to the results of the Beverly Allitt inquiry. *Nursing Times*, 92 (2) 23–25.

Manley, K. (2005) Transformational culture: a culture of effectiveness. Cited in McCormack, B., Manley, K. & Garbett, R. (eds) *Practice Development in Nursing.* Blackwell Publishing, Oxford.

Marquis, B.L. & Hutson, C.J. (2000) *Leadership Roles and Management Function in Nursing: Theory and Application*, 3rd edn. Lippincott, Philadelphia.

McSherry, R. (1999) Supporting patients and their families. In: *Caring for the Seriously Ill Patient* (C.C. Bassett & L. Mahin). Arnold, London.

McSherry, R. & Simmons, M. (2001) The importance of research dissemination and the barriers to implementation. In: *Evidence-Informed Nursing: A Guide for Clinical Nurses* (R. McSherry, M. Simmons & P. Abbott). Routledge, London.

McSherry, R., Simmons, M. & Abbott, P. (2001) *Evidence-Informed Nursing: A Guide for Clinical Nurses.* Routledge, London.

Mullally, S. (2001) Leadership and politics. *Nursing Management*, 8 (4) 21–27.

National Patient Safety Agency (2006) *Manchester Patient Safety Framework (MaPSaF).* http://www.npsa.nhs.uk/display?contentId=4798.

NHS Leadership Centre (2002) *NHS Leadership Qualities Framework.* http:// www.nhsleadershipqualities.nhs.uk/.

Northcott, N. (1999) Organizational effectiveness. *Nursing Times Learning Curve*, 3 (1) 10.

O'Neill, S. (2000) Clinical governance in action. Part 4: Communication. *Professional Nurse*, 16 (1) 816–817.

Parker, D. & Hudson, P. (2001) *Understanding Your Culture*. Shell International Exploration and Production, Rijswijk.

Phipps, K. (2000) Nursing and clinical governance. *British Journal of Clinical Governance*, 5 (2) 69–70.

Potter, A.P. & Perry, G.A. (1993) *Foundations of Nursing: Concepts, Process and Practice*. Mosby, London.

Ramsey, S. (2001) Audit exposes UK's worst serial killer. *The Lancet*, 357, 13 January, 123–124.

Scally, G. & Donaldson, L.J. (1998) Clinical governance and the drive for quality improvement in the new NHS in England. *BMJ*, 317, 61–65.

Squire, S. (2000) Clinical governance in action. Part 7: Effective learning. *Professional Nurse*, 16 (4) 1014–1015.

Stewart, R. (1996) *Leading in the NHS: A Practical Guide*, 2nd edn. Macmillan Business, London.

Westrum, R. (1992) Cultures with requisite imagination. In: *Verification and Validation of Complex Systems: Human Factors Issues* (eds J. Wise, D. Hopkin & P. Stager). Springer, Berlin, pp. 401–416.

Chapter 6

Clinical Governance and the Law

John Tingle

Introduction: defining terms

In focusing a legal discussion, lawyers are always keen to seek definitions of terms and to identify the parameters of discussion. Definitions and identification of parameters bring clarity and certainty. Clients can be advised where they stand and so can organise their affairs accordingly. Can this lawyer's exercise be usefully attempted with the term clinical governance? Is there one absolute definition that everyone subscribes to without exception and are there identifiable parameters to the topic?

On reading the literature, a number of definitions of the term do seem possible and the parameters of the topic do appear unclear. A lot can be seen to come under the term. In view of this fluidity of nature, it would seem appropriate to view clinical governance as one of those umbrella-type terms, like accountability, patient empowerment or lifelong learning. With these terms the focus is less on the term or label itself, and more on the ideas behind it. When the ideas behind the label are looked at, commonalities can often be seen to emerge. We have also seen the emergence of the term 'integrated governance', which draws the strands of a number of Government policy initiatives together including clinical governance. Integrated governance has been defined as (DH 2006):

> 'Integrated Governance is the means by which we pull together all the competing pressures on Boards and their supports (staff, advisors, systems and processes). It is a transitional position to good governance, but moves beyond the handling of issues in governance silos. It is clear that all healthcare organisations need to demonstrate that they have strengthened and streamlined their own governance arrangements and, over time, develop further integration between health and social care organisations in their health community.'

Clinical governance can be seen as a component part of integrated governance. From the perspective of the individual healthcarer, clinical governance would seem essentially to be about doing your job well, practising safely and reflectively, and helping to ensure the delivery of good quality healthcare and services.

Legal topics relevant to clinical governance could therefore range from health and safety law, employment law, ethical issues and dilemmas in medicine and nursing law, to consent, negligence, complaints, patient rights, patient safety, clinical risk management and so on. In fact, the legal discussion could be almost endless because of the fluid nature of the concept and the wide range of topics that can be encompassed within it.

In order to provide a reasoned legal treatment of relevant concepts, the discussion in this chapter will be focused on a selection of the topics mentioned above.

Litigation in the NHS

It is clear that the concept of clinical governance is being applied at a very difficult time in the NHS's history. Over the years litigation and complaints in the NHS have increased dramatically. The National Audit Office (2005) calculates the money owed by the NHS to patients injured by clinical negligence as follows (and see Fig. 6.1):

'However, over a number of years the NHS expects to pay out £7.8 billion (at today's prices) in respect of known or expected claims, after taking into account the likelihood of settlement of those claims. These sums are shown as provisions in the Authority's accounts. An additional £4.1 billion of claims are possible, but unlikely. These are shown as contingent liabilities in the Authority's accounts.'

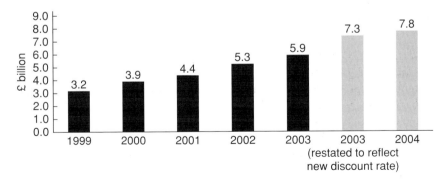

Fig. 6.1 Provisions for clinical negligence within the NHS (reproduced from National Audit Office/Audit Commission (2005) *Financial Management in the NHS*. The Stationery office, London.

The National Health Service Litigation Authority (2006) states:

'In 2004–05, 5,609 claims of clinical negligence and 3,766 claims of non-clinical negligence against NHS bodies were received by the NHSLA. This compares with 6,251 claims of clinical negligence and 3,819 claims of non-clinical negligence in 2003–04. £502.9 million was paid out in connection with clinical negligence claims in 2004–05. This figure includes both damages paid to patients and the legal costs borne by the NHS. In 2003–04, the comparable figure was £422.5 million. The figures for non-clinical claims are £25.1 million for 2004–05 and £10.1 million for 2003–04.'

Complaints to the Health Service Ombudsman (2004) increase every year:

'This year we have handled a higher workload than ever. We received a record 4,703 new complaints – an increase of 18% on the previous year, which had itself seen a huge rise in new complaints, many relating to continuing care.'

Almost every day stories appear in the press about medical mishaps, with patients being injured, though there is little evidence as to why they occur (Alberti 2001). This is, however, beginning to change as we receive such evidence through the work of the National Patient Safety Agency (NPSA). Criminal prosecutions by the Health and Safety Executive (HSE) against health bodies also reveal important failings in the provision of health services (HSE 2006). The notable medical scandals of Shipman, Alder Hey and Bristol have focused the public's attention and have put the medical profession on the defensive. Add to these scandals the increase in health litigation and complaints, and we have a serious 'lack of confidence problem' in the NHS to contend with. The Government and the NHS do, however, seem to have gained back some lost ground with a number of key patient-focused initiatives including the NHS Plan. The NHS Plan aimed to put patients at the centre of the NHS and worked from the clear premise that patients are the most important people in the health service (Tingle 2000). Subsequent to the NHS Plan organisational structures and initiatives have been developed to try to achieve a new patient centred NHS focus (DH, 2004, 2005a, b) and also to focus on how adverse incidents to patients occur and the development of strategies to avoid them. If successful, this activity will work to reduce the incidence of legal claims and complaints in the NHS and will hopefully bolster up patient confidence in the NHS.

The work of the NPSA and its National Reporting and Learning System (NRLS) is particularly notable in this area and their work is beginning to cast some light on why errors occur and what strategies can be adopted to make the NHS a safer place. The NPSA (2005) states:

'There were 85,342 incident reports to the National Reporting and Learning System (NRLS) between November 2003 and March 31 2005 affecting 86,142 patients. The majority of incidents – 68 per cent – resulted in no harm to patients and about one per cent led to severe harm or death. Reporting levels are increasing rapidly. Almost 75,000 reports were sent to the NRLS in the second quarter of the year between April and June. 230 Trusts reported to the NRLS during the period covered by the PSO report.'

Setting the scene

The former Health Secretary, Alan Milburn, set the scene for a patient focused NHS when he called for a new bond of trust between patients and the NHS (DH 2001) in a speech to patient groups at the King's Fund, London, on 29 January 2001. He stated:

'The NHS was conceived in an era of deference and hierarchy. The mantra that doctor knew best fitted the feel of the times. Those times have long since gone. But the NHS has lagged behind in its systems and in its culture, in the way it trains its staff and in the way it relates to its patients. We live in a different century. It is too much a 1940s system operating in a twenty-first century world.'

He called for a patient revolution in the NHS. The patient revolution he called for has only partially taken place, which is in itself a creditable occurrence. The old adage of 'aiming for the sky and hitting the tops of trees' comes to mind; the NHS is not yet fully patient focused and it must be a personal political judgment as to whether it ever will be. The NHS is a monolithic structure subject to too many competing agendas. It is also in an almost perpetual state of reform, which makes dramatic change impossible to achieve. The patient today is clearly more at the centre stage than when the first edition of this book appeared in 2002, thanks largely to the NHS Plan, but the competing issues, which seemed to weigh heavily on Trusts in 2002, have not gone away. Issues such as debt, the prudent use of limited financial resources and, very basically, just being able to manage to keep the structure intact and afloat on a day-to-day basis are still present despite record Government financial investment in the NHS. Today the NHS appears to be still largely reactive in management and policy style and in all fairness it cannot be regarded as being proactive; perhaps this is an inevitable fact of life, given its size and obligations.

Where are we now with clinical governance?

Clinical governance does function as a useful mechanism to help to refocus the NHS on being patient centred and it can also help reduce litigation and complaints by addressing clinical competence and patient safety issues. The work of the NPSA and NHSLA and the reports of the Healthcare Commission have also helped create a healthy momentum and focus in the NHS towards adopting strategies for a safer NHS. Progress is being made, albeit at a fairly slow and incremental pace. Regarding the achievements of clinical governance, the NAO (2003) states:

> 'NHS trusts acknowledged that the Controls Assurance and Clinical Negligence Scheme for Trusts and the performance (star) ratings have had beneficial impacts on their performance. But trusts assessed the Commission for Health Improvement clinical governance reviews as having the greatest impact on them. While they rarely reveal wholly new information about an organisation, they appear to have the effect of making knowledge about performance more explicit and visible, and thus stimulate meaningful changes in NHS trusts. However, many trusts' progress in implementing their Commission for Health Improvement action plans seems relatively slow. Strategic health authorities, which are now responsible for such follow-up, will need to ensure that trusts take timely action.'

The NAO (2005) also echoes these sentiments in regard to patient safety initiatives by stating:

> 'The safety culture within trusts is improving, driven largely by the Department's clinical governance initiative and the development of more effective risk management systems in response to incentives under initiatives such as the NHS Litigation Authority's Clinical Negligence Scheme for Trusts. . . . However, trusts are still predominantly reactive in their response to patient safety issues and parts of some organisations still operate a blame culture. All trusts have established effective reporting systems at the local level, although under-reporting remains a problem within some groups of staff, types of incidents and near misses.'

Progress is incremental and the NHS is a long way off from developing an ingrained patient safety culture, but it is certainly moving in the right direction; it has the correct infrastructure in place but the safety and governance messages have yet to permeate fully down to the staff in the workplace.

What is competent clinical practice?

A key component of effective clinical governance is that the risk of patient injury in the NHS is minimised and if possible completely eliminated. As a matter of common sense, if you practise competently, safely and reflectively the risks of adverse incidents will be much reduced and quality clinical practices maintained. It must, however, be recognised that it will not prove possible to totally eliminate error, given the complexity of modern NHS healthcare and the high numbers of patients being treated: according to the NAO (2005), 'every day over one million people are treated successfully by National Health Service (NHS) acute, ambulance and mental health trusts'.

The best that we can hope to do is to try to reduce the incidence of error as much as we can by practising competently and by managing risk effectively through an evidence base.

How the courts determine competent clinical practice

The law has a developed framework in the Tort of Negligence for dealing with competence issues, particularly where a patient claims to have been injured by a negligent conduct. This legal perspective is instructive because it provides an objective and authoritative assessment of the issues involved in competence assessment.

A court could be called upon to determine whether a doctor or nurse has been negligent. The term malpractice is sometimes used (Stauch *et al.* 2006):

> 'Medical malpractice may be defined, broadly, as any unjustified act or failure to act upon the part of a doctor or other health care worker which results in harm to the patient.'

In order to succeed in a malpractice action, the claimant or plaintiff (these words mean the same thing) must show that a legal duty of care existed towards the patient, that the duty was broken and that legally recognised harm was caused. For the purposes of this discussion the focus will be on the breach of duty.

A patient may complain, for example, that pressure sores were allowed to develop and were then not treated properly. There was no initial pressure sore risk assessment done and the sores just got worse. The patient has been off work for a number of weeks and this, he/she argues, could have been prevented had the nurse systematically assessed the patient for pressure sores and then treated them properly. The nurse, the patient argues, is in breach of his or her legal duty of care by not systematically assessing the patient, and then failing to treat the sores that developed. The nurse has behaved improperly and malpractice has occurred.

The word properly is important here. What is meant by this term? Lawyers would not necessarily know what proper treatment would be; they are not doctors or nurses, though some could well be. They would ask for an expert report from a leading wound care specialist and ask them, not what they would have done, but what they would have expected the ordinary skilled nurse in the relevant specialty to have done in the circumstances of the case. They need to determine the standard of care. The courts would not necessarily expect best practice but reasonable practice, though this is an issue of legal debate and conjecture.

Legally, competent, proper clinical practice is reasonable practice determined by reference to the famous *Bolam* case. Lord Browne-Wilkinson, in *Bolitho* v. *City and Hackney HA* [1998] Lloyds Rep Med 26 at 31, stated the following with regard to the standard of care and referred to *Bolam* thus:

'The locus classicus of the test for the standard of care required of a doctor or any other person professing some skill or competence is the direction to the jury given by McNair J in *Bolam* v. *Friern Hospital Management Committee* [1957] 1 WLR 583, 587.

I myself would prefer to put it this way, that he is not guilty of negligence if he has acted in accordance with a practice accepted as proper by a responsible body of medical men skilled in that particular art. Putting it the other way round, a man is not negligent, if he is acting in accordance with such a practice, merely because there is a body of opinion who would take a contrary view.'

Over the years the courts have been seen to be reluctant to challenge what experts have said about reasonable medical practices when assessing the standard of care, being unduly deferential to doctors, a theme made clear by Britain's most senior judge, the Lord Chief Justice, Lord Woolf (in a speech made in 2001):

'. . . until recently the courts treated the medical profession with excessive deference, but recently the position has changed. The over deferential approach is captured by the phrase "Doctor knows best". The contemporary approach is a more critical approach. It could be said to be that Doctor knows best if he acts reasonably and logically and gets his facts right.'

The courts can be seen to have adopted a more proactive approach to testing medical evidence and determining the standard of care. The *Bolitho* case is the baseline case for the new approach.

The case involved a two-year-old plaintiff who was re-admitted to hospital on 16 January 1984 after suffering a serious bout of the croup. On 17 January his condition deteriorated and there were two occasions where he had episodes of acute breathing problems. Twice the nurse observing him summoned the senior paediatric registrar but there was no response to the calls or from her senior house officer. The plaintiff suffered a third episode, which led to cardiac arrest and severe anoxic brain damage. It was accepted for the defendant that the failure of doctors to attend amounted to a breach of the duty of care. However, it was claimed that had they attended they would not have intubated.

'Although this was a defence based essentially on lack of causation, to succeed it required the court to accept that the hypothetical failure to intubate in such a case would not itself have been a breach of duty. In this regard, the defendant adduced evidence from a number of expert witnesses to the effect that, faced with a patient exhibiting the plaintiff's history and symptoms, they too would not intubate. The House of Lords agreed that the hypothetical decision not to intubate the plaintiff would have been in accord with responsible medical practice.' (Stauch *et al.* 2006)

The plaintiff lost his case. Lord Browne-Wilkinson stated the following:

'. . . in my view, the court is not bound to hold that a defendant doctor escapes liability for negligent treatment or diagnosis just because he leads evidence from a number of medical experts who are genuinely of opinion that the defendant's treatment or diagnosis accorded with sound medical practice. . . . The use of these adjectives – responsible, reasonable and respectable – all show that the court has to be satisfied that the exponents of the body of opinion relied upon can demonstrate that such opinion has a logical basis. In particular in cases involving, as they so often do, the weighing of risks against benefits, the judge before accepting a body of opinion as being responsible, reasonable, or respectable, will need to be satisfied that, in forming their views, the experts have directed their minds to the question of comparative risks and benefits and have reached a defensible conclusion on the matter.' (p. 33)

The *Bolitho* case reconsidered the *Bolam* test and placed it within context. *Bolam* has been returned to its proper limits and appropriate context, as Brazier and Miola (2000) conclude on the *Bolitho* decision:

> 'The decision does however signal judicial will, at the highest level, to return *Bolam* to its proper context. Together with the many other factors prompting change, inappropriate deference to medical opinion should be replaced by legal principles which recognise the imperative to listen to both doctors and patients and which acknowledge that the medical professional is just as much required to justify his or her practice as the architect or solicitor.'

The court's contemporary approach to determining the standard of care in medical malpractice can be regarded as an evidence-based approach, which fits in well with clinical governance and the new 'Patient Safety' focus in healthcare led by the NPSA. Foster (1998) feels that evidence-based medicine might begin to play a part in malpractice litigation after the *Bolitho* case:

> 'If the published evidence makes a wholly one-sided case against a particular medical practice, it will be difficult for any expert to say that its adoption by the defendant was reasonable, even though he or she is in august medical company in doing so.'

The Compensation Act 2006 makes it clear that, in considering what standard of care is reasonable in a claim for negligence or breach of statutory duty, courts can take into account whether requiring particular steps to be taken to meet the standard of care would prevent or impede a desirable activity from taking place. This provision is designed more broadly to attack 'the compensation culture perception' held by many, which can result in too much of a focus on risk management and so everyday activities suffer (schools banning conker matches, for example). There is also a provision which provides, in claims for negligence or breach of statutory duty, that an apology, offer of treatment or other redress shall not of itself amount to an admission of liability. Saying sorry does not mean you are admitting liability. An expression of regret suitably framed can avoid a complaint or even a legal claim.

The NHS Redress Bill currently proceeding through Parliament will affect the conduct of some lower value clinical negligence claims. Key measures of the Bill are the introduction of an NHS Redress Scheme to provide a speedy and appropriate response when something goes wrong and provide compensation where appropriate.

The law and clinical guidelines

Judges today will now be more influenced by national and local clinical guidelines issued by hospitals, NICE, the Royal Medical Colleges and other bodies that produce guidelines. This can be seen in the case of *Penney, Palmer and Cannon* v. *East Kent Health Authority* [2000] Lloyds Rep Med 41, discussed by Tingle and Rodgers (1999). This case concerned cervical smear tests and negligence allegations concerning interpretation of findings. Some slides had been labelled negatively when they should not have been and there was no medical follow-up for the claimants who subsequently went on to develop invasive adenocarcinoma of the cervix and had to undergo surgery, including a hysterectomy. Dismissing the Health Authority's appeal, the Court of Appeal held that because of the observable abnormalities on the slides they should not have been labelled negative. The standards of the CSP (cervical screening programme) were not complied with and consequently the Health Authority was liable in negligence. The trial judge had relied on a test of screener satisfaction known as 'the absolute confidence test', which according to the judge all the experts seemed to endorse. The trial judge had used this test in deciding the issue of the correct standard of care and whether this standard had been met. This test is incorporated into the clinical guidelines of the CSP.

This case shows clinical guidelines influencing judges and is a theme that should continue as NICE issues more guidelines.

The practice of evidence-based healthcare based on clinical guidelines is one way of demonstrating effective clinical governance. The courts would seem to support and use this approach in assessing whether malpractice has taken place or not. It could well be argued that reasonable clinical practice is no longer the acceptable judicial benchmark of appropriateness of clinical conduct. If most healthcarers are practising evidence-based best clinical practice, then surely the standard shifts from reasonable to best practice? In time cases will clarify this point.

Personal updating: knowledge and clinical guidelines

Professional staff development is an important aspect in demonstrating clinical governance and is the hallmark of a professional person. We would all expect professionals to keep up to date with changes and developments in their field of expertise. We rely on them and do not have the skill to second-guess them. In the healthcare context the expectations of professional updating are no different. It is possible that a malpractice case could be brought by a patient who argues that the doctor or nurse was negligent in not applying an appropriate clinical guideline, which would have helped them make a full recovery, or even some widely available research. A case could proceed on the basis of negligence through ignorance. A court would take the view that the reasonable doctor or nurse would be expected to keep up with professional developments in his or her sphere of practice, but what does this really entail? A doctor or nurse may read one article in the professional press about treating one condition and another may come out the following week advocating a different course of treatment. It is often said that medicine is not a science but a scientific-based art.

According to the present state of the law, minority medical or nursing opinion can still be *Bolam* reasonable with the caveat that the court will test the views. The courts will look for a logical basis and a risk benefit analysis. Clinical guidelines, nationally endorsed, may assist the court but may not be determinative. Each case will often depend on its own facts. Clinical guidelines do not suspend clinical autonomy. There is often more than one reasonable and logical way to care for a patient. A patient's condition may also contraindicate the application of the guideline or treatment. The healthcarer should always be prepared to advance a reasonable reason for not following the guideline or the usual course of treatment. Two cases assist on this issue.

In the case of *Crawford* v. *Board of Governors of Charing Cross Hospital* (*The Times*, 8 December 1953) the plaintiff developed brachial palsy as a result of his arm being kept in an extended position, at an angle of 80° from the body position, during an operation. Six months before, an article had appeared in *The Lancet* pointing out this danger. The anaesthetist had not read the article in question and the judge, Gerrard J., at first instance held the defendant liable for negligence. The Court of Appeal allowed the hospital's appeal and found the anaesthetist not negligent. Lord Denning stated that:

'. . . it would, I think, be putting too high a burden on a medical man to say that he has to read every article appearing in the current medical press; and it would be quite wrong to suggest that a medical man is negligent because he does not at once put into operation the suggestions which some contributor or other might make in a medical journal. The time may come in a particular case when a new recommendation may be so well proved and so well known, and so well accepted that it should be adopted, but that was not so in this case.'

Mason and Laurie (2005) comment:

'Failure to read a single article, it was said, may be excusable, while disregard of a series of warnings in the medical press could well be evidence of negligence. In view of the rapid progress currently being made in many areas of medicine, and in view of the amount of information confronting the average doctor, it is unreasonable to expect a doctor to be aware of every development in his field. At the same time, he must be reasonably up to date and must know of major developments. Hindsight is, of course, a harsh judge; yet in a number of HIV-related cases, the courts have indicated that doctors could not have been expected to have known of a risk at a time when its significance was only just being established. The practice of medicine has, however, become increasingly based on principles of scientific elucidation and report – the so-called 'evidence-based medicine' – and the pressure on doctors to keep abreast of current developments is now considerable. It is no longer possible for a doctor to coast along on the basis of long experience; such an attitude has been firmly discredited not only in medicine but in many other professions and callings.'

The views expressed by these authors are the views that courts would take today, though much would depend on the facts of the case in question. *Crawford* was a case in 1953; the information technology age is now firmly with us.

A more contemporary case on staff updating is *Gascoine* v. *Ian Sheridan and Co and Latham* [1994] 5 Med LR 437. This case concerned a number of issues, one of which was the responsibility of a consultant to keep informed about changes and developments in his specialty. Mitchell J. said that the consultant in the case was a very busy man 'who clearly had a responsibility to keep himself generally informed on mainstream changes in diagnosis treatment and practice through the mainstream literature such as the leading textbooks and *The Journal of Obstetrics and Gynaecology*'. The judge went on to say that it would be unreasonable for the consultant to 'acquaint himself with the content of the more obscure journals'.

A balance has to be drawn. The healthcarer should, at the very least, be prepared to demonstrate a systematic updating regime; just saying that you do not have the time to keep up to date is not enough. An awareness of the main clinical guidelines in the relevant specialty should also be demonstrated.

Good guidelines practice

We have seen that clinical guidelines can be used to convey evidence-based practice. Effective evidence-based practice demonstrates clinical governance in action. It is always good commonsense practice to date and sign a clinical guideline, and say who was involved in drafting it and what evidence was used. Always build in review dates. If you do not, how can you say that best practice is being followed? Practice changes, so a guideline should be reviewed. It is also worth stating on the guideline that the user must always use his or her own clinical judgement and that the guideline does not suspend this. These are commonsense steps, as guidelines could conceivably become the subject of legal actions. A patient could argue that a guideline was negligently designed and he/she has suffered as a result, or that another guideline should have been used. We have seen in the *Penney* case above how courts can treat guidelines. The DH also produces useful advice on using clinical guidelines (DH 1996) and identifies a number of legal considerations:

'(1) the objectives for the clinical guidelines need to be clear, and clearly stated. This will affect their subsequent legal standing;
(2) the intended use and applicability of clinical guidelines should be spelt out clearly, in the introduction;
(3) the guidelines must make clear for whom they are intended. The recommendations will usually be intended for a particular group of practitioners;
(4) clinical guidelines that no longer reflect best practice might conceivably become actionable, and developers need to incorporate specific statements about their validity and review procedure;
(5) they should be constructed in such a way that allows deviation and does not suffocate initiative that might bring about further improvements;
(6) the development of clinical guidelines must involve all the relevant professions and managers.'

This booklet provides lots of commonsense advice and should be read in conjunction with the advice offered on the NICE website (www.nice.org.uk). Guideline developers need to create in essence an audit trail of their work, as the information will prove useful in defending any claim of malpractice.

Conclusion

In conclusion, the law can be seen as an important mechanism to advance clinical governance. The courts are sensitive to the issues of evidence-based practice and the need to test clinical practice. Judges are not as deferential as they once were. Litigation and complaints are on the increase, but the Government can be seen to be developing key strategies to instil more confidence in the NHS. Clinical governance is just one tool being used; there are a number of others. The patient is to be viewed as king in the new NHS.

Professionals have a legal duty to keep up to date and cases have gone to court on this area. Clinical guidelines are an important quality development tool and a way of demonstrating the existence of the practice of evidence-based care and the operation of clinical governance. The courts remain the final arbiters of what is acceptable clinical practice and they are the ultimate and final mechanism of clinical accountability.

Suggested reading

Eccles, M. & Grimshaw, J. (eds) (2000) *Clinical Guidelines From Conception to Use*. Radcliffe Medical Press, Oxford.

Furrow, B.R. (1999) Broadcasting clinical guidelines on the internet: will physicians tune in? *American Journal of Law and Medicine*, 25 (2 and 3) 403–421.

Garwood-Gowers Austin, Tingle J. & Wheat, K. (2005) *Contemporary Issues in Healthcare Law and Ethics*. Butterworth Heinemann, Oxford.

Tingle, J., Foster, C. & Wheat, K. (eds) (2004) *Regulating Healthcare Quality, Legal and Professional Issues*. Butterworth Heinemann, Oxford.

References

Alberti, K.G.M.M. (2001) Medical errors: a common problem. *BMJ*, 322, 3 March, 501.

Brazier, M. & Miola, J. (2000) Bye-bye *Bolam*: a medical litigation revolution? *Medical Law Review*, 8 (1) Spring, 85–114.

Department of Health (1996) *Clinical Guidelines, Using Clinical Guidelines to Improve Patient Care Within the NHS*. DH, London.

Department of Health (2001) *A new bond of trust between patients and the NHS*. Alan Milburn speech to patient groups at the King's Fund, Monday 29 January 2001. DH Press Release 2001/0057. DH, London.

Department of Health (2004) *The NHS Improvement Plan: Putting People at the Heart of Public Services*. DH, London.

Department of Health (2005a) *Creating a Patient-Led NHS: Delivering the NHS Improvement Plan*. DH, London.

Department of Health (2005b) *Health Reform in England: Update and Next Steps*. DH, London.

Department of Health (2006) *Integrated Governance Handbook*. DH, London.

Foster, C. (1998) *Bolam*: consolidation and clarification. *Health Care Risk Report*, 4 (5) April 5–7.

Health and Safety Executive (2006) *HSE Public Register of Convictions*. HSE, London. www.hse-databases.co.uk/prosecutions.

Health Service Ombudsman (2004) *Annual Report 2003–04, HC703*. The Stationery Office, London.

Mason, J.K. & Laurie, G.T. (2005) *Mason and McCall Smith's Law and Medical Ethics*, 7th edn. Oxford University Press, London.

National Audit Office (2003) *Achieving Improvements Through Clinical Governance: A Progress Report on Implementation by NHS Trusts*. HC 1055. The Stationery Office, London.

National Audit Office (2005) *A Safer Place for Patients: Learning to Improve Patient Safety*. The Stationery Office, London.

National Audit Office/Audit Commission (2005) *Financial Management in the NHS*. The Stationery Office, London.

National Health Service Litigation Authority (2006) *About the NHS Litigation Authority*. NHSLA, London. www.nhsla.com.

National Patient Safety Agency (2005) *Building a memory: preventing harm, reducing risks and improving patient safety*. The first report of the National Reporting and Learning System and the Patient Safety Observatory, July 2005. NPSA, London.

Stauch, M. & Wheat, K. with Tingle, J.H. (2006) *Text, Case and Materials on Medical Law*, 3rd edn. Routledge Cavendish, Oxford.

Tingle, J.H. (2000) The new, ambitious NHS Plan. *Health Care Risk Report*, 6 (10) October 23–24.

Tingle, J.H. & Rodgers, M.E. (1999) Clinical guidelines, NICE and the Court of Appeal. *Nottingham Law School Journal*, 8 (2).

Chapter 7

The Impact of Clinical Governance in the National Health Service

Rob McSherry and Paddy Pearce

Introduction

The chapter will explore the empirical and contemporary literature to demonstrate the impact of clinical governance at an individual, team and organisational level. The relative merits and demerits of clinical governance will be debated.

Clinical governance: friend or foe?

When clinical governance was introduced into the NHS in 1997 (DH 1997) there was a degree of cynicism about its ability to achieve its goals because healthcare professionals were divided in their opinions:

> 'The subject is one which divides doctors [indeed all healthcare professionals] into two groups. The minority believe that clinical governance will prove to be a useful tool for introducing quality improvements into health care, whereas the majority consists of those cynics who believe the topic is another "flavour of the month" which will go away if ignored.' (Gaminara 2000, p. 80)

Dependent on your viewpoint, clinical governance was either embraced or resisted. Whilst acknowledging the range of views from the cynics to the optimists, clinical governance has unfortunately or fortunately begun to be accepted as part of the NHS culture of today. As Halligan suggests, clinical governance is here to stay: 'The brand with its implicit promise of patient-centred, accountable care has put down roots in our healthcare culture. Despite the initial perceptions of threat and challenge to organisational and clinical autonomy sometimes flagged up by the phrase, it has become part of the vernacular of the NHS' (Halligan 2006, p. 6). Whilst agreeing with Halligan's view, we would suggest this needs to be substantiated with the backing of empirical evidence. The notion of demonstrating the impact of clinical governance is imperative given the fact that its principles have transcended into almost all healthcare disciplines; for instance, dentistry, pharmacy, prison healthcare services, Primary Care Trusts, the independent sector, to name but a few. The concept seems to have permeated from the hierarchy of boards to the grass roots where clinical practice occurs. However, what evidence is available to justify its relative merits and demerits to individuals, teams and organisations?

A literature search on Google highlighted over 1.6 million hits associated with clinical governance, demonstrating its popularity across the globe. Similarly the various healthcare databases such as CINHAL and MEDLINE reveal a proliferation of literature defining the key components and associated issues of clinical governance within the healthcare setting. However, a critical review and synthesis of this literature illustrates minimal empirical-based studies demonstrating the impact of clinical governance.

Revealing the impact of clinical governance

The impact of clinical governance is emerging through the undertaking of empirical-based evaluation studies. However, we would like to acknowledge that this is not a systematic review or indeed an in-depth critical review of all the empirical studies available. It is our intention to raise awareness of the importance of focusing on evaluating the impact of clinical governance. We believe this is imperative given the significant amount of finances and resources invested in implementing clinical governance, which according to the National Audit Office (NAO) was estimated to cost the NHS approximately £60 million in 2002–2003 (NAO 2003, p. 4). A critical review of five studies by Hartley *et al.* (2002), Degeling *et al.* (2003), NAO (2003), Freeman and Walshe (2004), and Wallace *et al.* 2004) (see Table 7.1) provides some evidence to demonstrate the impact of clinical governance at national and regional level. It is evident that clinical governance is making a difference in the following five key areas: accountability, organisational structures, continuous quality improvement, performance management and culture. The remainder of this section will focus on highlighting how clinical governance has influenced these areas both positive and negatively.

Accountability

The Freeman and Walshe (2004) study reported that clinical governance has played a major role in highlighting and improving corporate accountability

Table 7.1 Research studies reporting on the impact of clinical governance (in chronological order).

Study: Freeman, T. & Walshe, K. (2004) Achieving progress through clinical governance, a national study of healthcare managers' perception in the NHS in England
Origin: England
Purpose: To explore the perception of progress made with clinical governance
Method: Quantitative method using the Organisational Progress in Clinical Governance (OPCG) schedule
Sample: Random sample ($n = 100$). Board members and directorate managers of English acute, mental health/learning difficulties trusts
Main findings:
- Evidence that structures for clinical governance are established
- More progress has been made with assurance and corporate accountability
- Progress is less advanced in quality improvement, leadership and collaborative working
- Managers' perceptions of achievement were slightly lower than those of board members

Study: Wallace, L.M., Boxall, M. & Spurgeon, P. (2004) Organisational change through clinician governance: the West Midlands three years on
Origin: England
Purpose: To examine the perception of clinical governance leads 2.5 years after a baseline assessment
Method: Survey using semistructured telephone interviews
Sample: All 40 NHS Trusts in the West Midlands, England
Main findings:
- Expected outcomes were achieved more often than expected at the time of the baseline assessment
- Improved patient outcomes and documented changes in clinical behaviour were expected and achieved
- A more open culture was evident in 84% of Trusts
- A new approach to consultant appraisal and critical incidents was welcomed
- League tables and external review had an adverse effect where results were poor; however, where results were positive the impact was small

---

Table 7.1 *(cont'd)*

Study: Degeling, P., Maxwell, K.J., Coyle, B. & MacBeth, F. (2003) The impact of CHI: evidence from Wales
Origin: Wales
Purpose:
Method: Survey and focus groups
Sample: Six Welsh Trusts
Main findings:
- CHI's Clinical Governance Reviews seem to have had little impact on the NHS
- For CHI to be more effective it needs to move away from assessing the seven pillars of clinical governance
- Healthcare professionals have different experiences with understanding evaluations of clinical governance
- Each professional group seems to be influenced by its professional culture
- CHI needs to increase its awareness of how grass roots clinical staff perceive and evaluate clinical governance
- CHI needs to provide a very clear message about the specific changes in practice and culture it is seeking to achieve

Study: National Audit Office (2003) Achieving improvement through clinical governance: a progress report on implementation by NHS Trusts
Origin: England
Purpose: To provide the UK government with an independent assessment of progress made with the implementation of clinical governance
Method:
- A census of the NHS Trust
- Survey of board members and senior managers
- Review of reports from CHI
- Interviews with the DH and regional staff
Sample: A combined total of 100 Acute NHS Trusts, Mental Health Trusts and Ambulance Trusts
Main findings:
- Implementation of clinical governance has raised the profile quality issues for boards of NHS Trusts
- Virtually all NHS Trusts have laid the necessary foundations, but all the components of clinical governance are fully embedded in all clinical directorates
- The implementation of clinical governance between and within Trusts is patchy
- There is greater accountability for clinical performance in Trusts
- There has been a change in clinical culture becoming more transparent
- There is evidence of more collaborative working

Table 7.1 *(cont'd)*

- There is evidence of improvements in practice and patient care, yet Trusts still require robust processes for measuring overall progress
- There remains room for improvement with:
  - ○ The provision of support for the implementation of clinical governance
  - ○ Communication between NHS boards and clinical directorates
  - ○ The development of a coherent approach to quality improvement, processes for risk management and performance management and the systematic dissemination of sharing lessons learnt with the rest of the NHS
- Where NHS Trusts have been more successful with the implementation of clinical governance the key features identified were:
  - ○ Strong leadership
  - ○ Commitment to staff
  - ○ Willingness to consider doing things differently

Study: Hartley, A.M., Griffiths, R.K. & Saunders, K.L. (2002) An evaluation of clinical governance in the public health departments of the West Midlands Region to assess two models for examining clinical governance in public health – namely the model produced by the Faculty of Public Health and the West Midlands SPOCK model

Origin: England

Purpose: To evaluate the development of clinical governance in public health departments

Method: Semi-structured interviews carried out during the annual visit by the regional director of public health

Sample: All Health Authorities in the West Midlands region. Directors of public health

Main findings:

- Both models were useful in examining clinical governance
- A combination of both models produced better results
- The West Midlands public health department valued annual visits as they provided external peer review
- Public health departments have ownership of the process
- Most departments felt that clinical governance provided a framework to bring together a range of existing governance activities into a more coherent whole
- Appraisal and CPD were well addressed
- Half of the departments reported good resource allocation for clinical governance
- Nine departments felt that clinical governance had a high organisational profile

structures within NHS Trusts. Corporate accountability in this instance referred to the efficiency and effectiveness of NHS boards, committees and associated systems and processes for managing and dealing with clinical risks or quality related issues. Whilst it is evident that significant progress has been made in changing attitudes at executive and board levels, Freeman and Walshe's (2004) study revealed a difference in the perception of progress between managers and directors. Similarly the NAO (2003) study concluded that clinical governance has raised the profile of quality issues for corporate boards, yet there remains a degree of inconsistency between and within the various NHS organisations. The Hartley *et al.* (2002) study provides some insight into the impact of clinical governance relating to the importance of accountability via continued professional development (CPD), appraisal and personal development plans (PPD) at an individual level. The findings from Hartley et al. (2002), NAO (2003) and Freeman and Walshe (2004) demonstrate that clinical governance has raised the profile of quality for NHS boards. Further work needs to be done to highlight and embed the importance of accountability at a team and individual level. This will only be achieved by having robust systems and processes in place that are adequately and appropriately resourced and managed.

Organisational structures

The NAO (2003) reported that the majority of NHS organisations have the necessary clinical governance foundations, although these are not fully embedded in clinical directorates: 'Clinical governance is well established and embedded in the corporate systems of the vast majority of NHS Trusts, with board level executive and non-executive leadership, trust wide committee structures, and a strong executive function in the form of a clinical governance department or unit' (NAO 2003, p. 4). Wallace *et al.* (2004) like NAO (2003) highlighted the importance of having the necessary clinical governance systems and processes in place to ensure and improve quality. Similarly, Freeman and Walshe (2004) found that clinical governance 'structures seem to be well established' within the NHS Trusts surveyed. However, we would argue that whilst the necessary structures are in place for the implementation of clinical governance, healthcare professionals and support staff need to be made aware of what these structures are, how they function and what benefits they provide to both the organisation and individuals themselves. Furthermore, we would suggest that the development of any clinical governance systems and processes should involve and ultimately benefit patients, carers and the public they serve. Continuous quality improvement will not be achieved without having the necessary structures in place.

Continuous quality improvement

All the studies identified how clinical governance has influenced the quality improvement agenda. The NAO (2003) noted that there have been improvements in practice and patient care. However, this has been undertaken in an unsystematic and ad hoc manner and requires further attention and developments to ensure this becomes systematic in the future. Freeman and Walshe (2004) like NAO (2003) found that progress with quality improvement was less advanced than other aspects of clinical governance included in their study, for instance corporate accountability and risk management. Wallace *et al.* (2004) reported improvements in patient care following the introduction of clinical governance by around 80% from the initial baseline measure. This finding reinforces the need for advancing clinical governance frameworks within all NHS organisations. Degeling *et al.* (2003), unlike the Freeman and Walshe (2004) and NAO (2003) evaluation studies which targeted organisational aspects of clinical governance, focused on highlighting the impact of clinical governance reviews on practice. Six Welsh Trusts were involved where a combination of surveys and focus group interviews were undertaken to elicit healthcare staffs' perspectives regarding clinical governance reviews. The study concluded that the impact of CHI reviews had minimal impact on the quality improvement agenda. The Hartley *et al.* (2002) study of public health departments in the West Midlands region of England noted the positive effects of clinical governance surrounding CPD, appraisal and life-long learning and how these factors ultimately influence quality of care and services.

Taking the empirical evidence provided by Degeling *et al.* (2003), NAO (2003), Freeman and Walshe (2004), and Wallace *et al.* (2004) into account it would be reasonable to suggest that clinical governance has played a major role in advancing and embedding the concept of continuous quality improvement within NHS organisations. Further work on engaging, empowering, enlightening and encouraging all staff working in clinical and non-clinical teams delivering patient care and services is essential. As continuous quality improvement as reported by Freeman and Walshe (2004) has had a major impact on patient experience and patient outcome we are in agreement with the authors of this report that further work to involve patients, users and the public is vital.

Performance management

Performance management emerges indirectly as a key feature of clinical governance in the way quality improvement is targeted and measured. The majority of these studies allude to the need for a systematic approach to performance management in order to detect changes both positive and negative with service and practice developments. Since the introduction of clinical governance within the NHS we have witnessed many improvements in healthcare, including reductions in waiting times for elective procedures and outpatient appointments (DH 2005), improvements in treatments and outcomes, the adoption of evidence-based healthcare, improvements in clinical risk management and patient safety systems, the emergence of an open culture of learning, and greater involvement of patients and the public in the planning, provision, delivery and evaluation of services. However, the evidence thus far is limited in confirming how these important changes in service provision have made a difference.

The impact of clinical governance in our opinion has provided NHS boards of healthcare organisations, managers and healthcare professionals with a framework that has harmonised two seemingly contrasting concepts: that of performance management and quality improvement. Performance management, defined as 'the process of quantifying the efficiency and effectiveness of purposeful action and decision-making' (Waggoner *et al.* 1999), is an integral part of successful modernisation. According to McSherry and Pearce (2002) this is because performance management involves developing, implementing and evaluating a series of complex systems and processes that detect good and not so good practice of either devices or personnel. Garland (1998) argues that performance management is about the integration of various systems and sources of reported information in highlighting the overall quality status of the organisation. By combining the Waggoner *et al.* (1999) and McSherry and Pearce (2002) works with the empirical study provided by Hartley *et al.* (2002) it is evident that Individual Performance Review (IPR) and Team Action Planning (TAP) play a fundamental role in achieving quality services within performance management frameworks. This is because successful implementation of clinical governance is dependent on the level of organisational, team and individual engagement with and in the various systems and processes. Performance management and continuous quality improvement collectively are about making and sustaining changes to improve the systems and processes which will ultimately impact on the patients' outcomes.

The concept of quality improvement is dear to the heart of most healthcare professionals because we all want the best for our patients and service users. Strange at it sounds to some, the vast majority of healthcare managers also want to improve patient care and services. Yet, the empirical studies provided suggest that the development of robust systems and processes of continuous quality improvement and performance management is dependent on the organisational culture and working environment in which we work.

Culture

Culture emerges from the reported studies as a key contributor to the successful implementation and continued success of clinical governance. Returning to the DH (1997) original definition of clinical governance – 'a framework through which NHS organisations are accountable for continuously improving the quality of their services and safeguarding high standards of care by creating an environment in which clinical excellence will flourish' – it is evident that clinical governance is undoubtedly emerging as a major framework for sustaining, assuring, developing and demonstrating excellence in practice. Based on the findings from the evaluation studies, the creation of an environment in which clinical excellence will flourish is about creating and nurturing an open culture of learning and facilitation where CPD and lifelong learning are valued and patients are placed at centre stage of all we do. The majority of the studies included in this brief literature review make either direct or indirect reference to organisational culture and change as major players in achieving successful governance. The NAO (2003) noted that there has been a change in clinical culture, which is becoming more transparent. Degeling *et al.* (2003) note that healthcare professionals have different experiences with understanding evaluations of clinical governance, where each professional group seems to be influenced by its professional culture and efforts need to be made to increase awareness of how grass roots clinical staff perceive and evaluate clinical governance.

Recipe for successes

To successfully develop an organisational culture that values clinical governance, several key factors emerge. The evidence to date suggests that to successfully develop a framework of clinical governance that ultimately impacts on the provision of excellence in practice is dependent on several factors:

- Strong leadership: leadership is required at all levels of the organisation, resonating from the top of the organisation to staff working in all areas of the organisation. Where possible the development of shared governance or self-governing teams should be nurtured in avoiding the stereotypical hierarchical approach to managing and leading change. Senior managers, clinicians and leaders of services need to lead by example and be committed for the course.
- Support and resources: from all staff working in the NHS and financial resourcing and backing; these need to be provided in order to realise the full potential that clinical governance can provide. The various

departments and associated systems and processes all need to communicate efficiently and effectively in order to realise the benefits that interdependency and collaborative working can provide.

- Culture: the creation of an honest, open and transparent culture, where things that go wrong or not so well are viewed in the light of a just blame culture where learning is at the heart of the organisation. This proactive as opposed to reactive approach to management and leadership is paramount to the successful implementation and continued development of clinical governance.
- CPD and lifelong learning: these are imperative to ensure that all staff have the necessary knowledge, skills and confidence to perform their roles and responsibilities in a competent, efficient and effective way. Lifelong learning should be seen as the norm, where staff are willing to do things differently.

Conclusion

The empirical evidence to date reveals that the key critical success factors of clinical governance can be categorised into five key areas: accountability, organisational structures, continuous quality improvement, performance management and culture. Despite these initial findings, much more empirical-based evaluation is needed in order to confirm or refute the impact of clinical governance. A limitation of these studies is the fact that they are primarily focused on secondary care rather than primary care or a combination of both. We would echo Halligan's (2006, p. 7) words: 'what we have learnt, more than anything else, is that if clinical governance gains purchase in the hearts and minds of frontline staff and is built up from the bottom, then the strength of that frontline mandate is unstoppable'. The challenge is in acquiring the resources to engage frontline staff in taking ownership to continually drive clinical governance forward in their local context and setting.

Key points

- Dependent on your viewpoint, clinical governance will be either embraced or resisted.
- The impact of clinical governance is emerging through the undertaking of empirical-based evaluation studies.
- Clinical governance has played a major role in highlighting and improving corporate accountability structures within NHS Trusts, but more work needs to be done to ensure the same for individuals.

- The development of any clinical governance system and process should involve and ultimately benefit patients, carers and the public they serve.
- Performance management and continuous quality improvement collectively is about making and sustaining changes to improve the systems and processes, which will ultimately impact on the patients' outcomes.
- Based on the findings from the evaluation studies, the creation of an environment in which clinical excellence will flourish is about creating and nurturing an open culture of learning and facilitation where CPD and lifelong learning are valued and patients are placed at centre stage of all we do.

Suggested reading

Degeling, P., Maxwell, S., Kennedy, J., Coyle, B. & MacBeth, F. (2003) The impact of CHI: evidence from Wales. *Quality in Primary Care*, 11 (2) 147–154.

Department of Health (1997) *The New NHS: Modern, Dependable*. The Stationery Office, London.

Freeman, T. & Walshe, K. (2004) Achieving progress through clinical governance? A national study of healthcare managers' perception in the NHS in England. *Quality and Safety in Healthcare*, 13, 335–343.

Hartley, M., Griffiths, R.K. & Saunders, K.L. (2002) An evaluation of clinical governance in the public health departments of the West Midlands region. *Journal of Epidemiology and Community Health*, 56, 563–568.

National Audit Office (2003) *Achieving Improvements Through Clinical Governance: A Progress Report on Implementation by NHS Trusts*. National Audit Office, London.

Wallace, L.M., Boxall, M. & Spurgoen, P. (2004) Organisational change through clinical governance. *Clinical Governance: An International Journal*, 9 (1), 17–30.

References

Department of Health (1997) *The New NHS: Modern, Dependable*. The Stationery Office, London.

Degeling, P., Maxwell, S., Kennedy, J., Coyle, B. & MacBeth, F. (2003) The impact of CHI: evidence from Wales. *Quality in Primary Care*, 11 (2) 147–154.

Freeman, T. & Walshe, K. (2004) Achieving progress through clinical governance? A national study of healthcare managers' perception in the NHS in England. *Quality and Safety in Healthcare*, 13, 335–343.

Gaminara, E.J. (2000) Book review of *Clinical Governance: Making it Happen* (M. Lugon & J. Secker-Walker). Royal Society of Medicine. *Quality in Health Care*, 9, 80.

Garland, G. (1998) Governance. *Nursing Management*, 56, 28–31.

Halligan, A. (2006) Clinical governance: assuring the sacred duty of trust to patients. *Clinical Governance: An International Journal*, 11 (1) 5–7.

Hartley, M., Griffiths, R.K. & Saunders, K.L. (2002) An evaluation of clinical governance in the public health departments of the West Midlands region. *Journal of Epidemiology and Community Health*, 56, 563–568.

McSherry, R. & Pearce, P. (2002) Clinical Governance: A Guide to Implementation for Healthcare Professionals. Blackwell Science, Oxford.

National Audit Office (2003) *Achieving Improvements Through Clinical Governance. A Progress Report on Implementation by NHS Trusts*. National Audit Office, London.

Waggoner, D.B., Neeley, A.D. & Kennerley, N.P. (1999) The forces that shape organisational performance management systems: an interdisciplinary view. *International Journal of Production Economics*, 53–60, 60–61.

Wallace, L.M., Boxall, M. & Spurgoen, P. (2004) Organisational change through clinical governance. *Clinical Governance: An International Journal*, 9 (1), 17–30.

Chapter 8

Conclusion: The Future of Clinical Governance for Healthcare Professionals

Rob McSherry and Paddy Pearce

In this second edition we have described why clinical governance is needed and what it is, together with its key components and how they relate to practising clinicians, teams and organisations. The challenge for some healthcare organisations, teams and individuals, according to Professor Halligan (cited in the *Financial Times* 2006), remains in resolving the barriers, and keeping abreast of current healthcare reform and policy in order for the successful implementation of clinical governance. For example, the current financial deficit facing the NHS organisation has led to job cuts and service reviews. We believe these changes have affected staff morale and may ultimately have a direct and detrimental effect on patient experience and continuous quality improvement, making it imperative for individuals, teams and organisations to keep up to date with the law, as outlined in Chapter 6.

Given the importance with which the current government and no doubt future governments regard clinical governance, it goes without saying that the concept is here to stay. Some authors would argue that 'integrated governance' should replace that of clinical governance. We would echo the desirability of healthcare governance, which acknowledges the interdependency of the various faces of governance in integrating the various components of governance; for example, corporate, clinical, research, etc. However, we believe that clinical governance should remain independent but an integral part of the integrated governance framework because it is a concept or set of systems and processes that clinicians and managers are beginning to embrace. To shift the focus of clinical governance away to that of integrated governance too quickly may ultimately have a detrimental effect on clinical staffs' perceptions of governance and lead to disengagement rather than continuing to engage with the term in the future.

The desire of healthcare professionals and the public alike for the continuous improvement in clinical quality, in striving for excellence, further reinforces the need for clinical governance. Over the past 52 years we have witnessed many changes in the NHS, where some seem to have introduced 'changing things for the sake of change'. The changes attributed to clinical governance are somewhat different and cannot be viewed by the cynics as alluded to by Baker (2000) – the change for change's sake approach to healthcare policy – because clinical governance is a broad framework that has encompassed many different strands of quality under a collective umbrella and made leaders of healthcare organisations responsible and accountable for assuring clinical and non-clinical quality.

We continue to be convinced even in such difficult and challenging times that clinical governance provides NHS organisations, teams and individuals with a golden opportunity to make genuine and lasting improvements in the systems and process of care delivery as managerial and clinical responsibilities are harmonised.

The real opportunities and challenges facing some healthcare organisations, teams and individuals are in the development of realistic and achievable strategies that support their quest for the continuous quality improvement in providing excellent clinical care. Organisations, teams and individuals that are truly committed to clinical governance will realise that clinical governance is everybody's business, by ensuring a multidisciplinary and multiagency approach to the development of future services. For clinical governance to realise its potential the concept as part of the AfC should be written into all job descriptions and contracts of employment for all NHS employees, an approach that reinforces the concept of ensuring accountability by all NHS staff for the provision of high quality care. Clinical governance must be included in the induction of all employees in ensuring a move towards the development, implementation and evaluation of the care, treatment or interventions they provide. A culture of openness, honesty and transparency with a willingness to learn from mistakes and share good and not so good practices needs to become the norm. The creation of such a culture requires time, commitment, vision, ambition and patience over a long period, where good communications, collaborations and partnerships between and within the systems and processes akin to clinical governance, along with the professions, are fundamental (Donaldson 2000).

The challenge for the future of healthcare is in resolving the barriers to clinical governance, barriers that are related to the founding principles of the NHS in ensuring universal access to a comprehensive service based on clinical need, where equity, diversity and equality of the services will be assured for all. These principles can only be assured in an organisation that is open to criticism and learns from its mistakes, as the recent media attention continues to inform the NHS. To ensure this open culture where expressing one's concerns or celebrating success becomes the norm, management and leadership that are transformational and democratic in nature requires development, where staff are valued and developed through the instigation of mutual partnerships, shared decision-making and ownership that reinforces the concept of accountability via the clinical governance framework.

The task for individual healthcare professionals is in developing their knowledge, understanding and skills of applying the concept of clinical governance to their daily practice. Aligning clinical governance alongside their personal and professional development plans and KSF can only serve the professional well in the future. However, this will only become effective in an organisation that proactively seeks and values the true potential that clinical governance can unlock for its own organisation. Genuine sustained support and commitment needs to be guaranteed from the boards to the shop floor. The National Plan 2000 clearly stated and stipulated the need for the adoption of a clinical governance framework by the organisation, team and individual by basing the entire document around assuring the continuous quality improvements of the NHS – a quality service that will be measured and evaluated against set national standards of care derived from the best available evidence published by NICE. The adherence to these standards along with the implementation of the clinical governance framework continues to be assessed and reviewed by the HC, which should be viewed as a supporting not a policing agency in evolving the future of the NHS.

We believe that as healthcare professionals concerned with providing the best standards of care to our patients, carers, service users and the public we need to continually embrace this wonderful opportunity to partake in the reformation of our NHS. Clinical governance remains a vehicle to enable us to do this efficiently and effectively. So let us get involved with clinical governance in making a real and lasting difference for our NHS and patients in our care.

Good luck!

References

Baker, M. (2000) *Making Sense of the NHS White Papers*, 2nd edn. Radcliffe Medical Press Ltd, Oxford.

Donaldson, L.J. (2000) Clinical governance; a mission to improve. *British Journal of Clinical Governance*, 5 (1), 6–8.

Halligan, A. (2006) Quoted in Real Reform of Health Service 'a Deceit' (N. Timmins). *Financial Times*, 3 April. http://www.reform.co.uk/website/pressroom/articles.aspx?o=233

Index